About Island Press

Since 1984, the nonprofit organization Island Press has been stimulating, shaping, and communicating ideas that are essential for solving environmental problems worldwide. With more than 1,000 titles in print and some 30 new releases each year, we are the nation's leading publisher on environmental issues. We identify innovative thinkers and emerging trends in the environmental field. We work with world-renowned experts and authors to develop cross-disciplinary solutions to environmental challenges.

Island Press designs and executes educational campaigns, in conjunction with our authors, to communicate their critical messages in print, in person, and online using the latest technologies, innovative programs, and the media. Our goal is to reach targeted audiences—scientists, policy makers, environmental advocates, urban planners, the media, and concerned citizens—with information that can be used to create the framework for long-term ecological health and human well-being.

Island Press gratefully acknowledges major support from The Bobolink Foundation, Caldera Foundation, The Curtis and Edith Munson Foundation, The Forrest C. and Frances H. Lattner Foundation, The JPB Foundation, The Kresge Foundation, The Summit Charitable Foundation, Inc., and many other generous organizations and individuals.

The opinions expressed in this book are those of the author(s) and do not necessarily reflect the views of our supporters.

Grain by Grain

Grain by Grain

A QUEST TO REVIVE ANCIENT WHEAT, RURAL JOBS, AND HEALTHY FOOD

Bob Quinn and Liz Carlisle

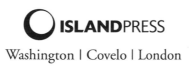

ISLANDPRESS

Washington | Covelo | London

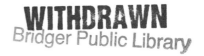

ISLAND PRESS is a trademark of the Center for Resource Economics.

Library of Congress Control Number: 2018961749

All Island Press books are printed on environmentally responsible materials.

Manufactured in the United States of America
10 9 8 7 6 5 4 3 2 1

Keywords: Kamut; organic; gluten sensitivity; heirloom grains; ancient wheat; regenerative farming; sustainable agriculture; pesticides; Big Sandy, Montana; local food; rural economy

Contents

Prologue
Liz Carlisle

I arrived on Capitol Hill in June 2008, a fresh-faced young staffer determined to change the world. I had spent the past four years touring the American heartland as a country singer, witnessing the economic pain of rural communities in decline. Wishing I could do more to help, I'd been inspired by an organic farmer from my home state of Montana who had recently unseated a three-term incumbent to win election to the United States Senate. His name was Jon Tester, and I was now his legislative correspondent for agriculture and natural resources.

As a Montana native, I understood that many of our constituents were wary of the federal government's involvement in these matters. More than a quarter of the population earned their living in agriculture, mining, or construction. Many of these people felt left behind by shifts in the global economy and were vehemently opposed to any regulation that might make their livelihoods even more tenuous.

My first week on the job, I was told that my task would be to record and respond to emails about my issue areas, to ensure the senator was informed about constituents' views. "In this office," our legislative director told me, "we still believe that the best ideas come from citizens."

Excited, but a bit overwhelmed by the breadth of topics about which I needed to become knowledgeable, I was relieved when my supervisor introduced me to Matt Jennings, the legislative assistant handling agriculture, energy, and natural resources. Matt had been working for Jon since the senator was a state legislator, and he was a walking encyclopedia about everything from the details of pending legislation to which agency staffers were long talkers. As I quickly learned, Matt liked to get to the point, and he wasn't afraid to cut off a windbag lobbyist or break with Capitol Hill protocol to do so. One day, tired of waiting on the work order process that ensued whenever the heating unit malfunctioned in our old office in the Russell Building, Matt whipped out a Swiss Army knife that he'd somehow gotten through security and proceeded to tinker with it himself.

Taking the same can-do, do-it-yourself approach to policy, Matt tipped me off to the salt-of-the-earth geniuses of our state, from the rancher-led coalition restoring a watershed burdened by the toxic legacy of mining to the network of heirloom lentil farmers with whom I would eventually collaborate on my PhD dissertation. One day, when I popped over to his workstation unannounced with a burning question about the viability of renewable energy in Montana, he answered, as he often did, with a name instead of a number. "Bob Quinn," Matt said, pulling up a news story about Montana's first wind farm, which had started harvesting power a few years earlier near the little town of Judith Gap. I leaned over Matt's computer to get a better look at a man in a cowboy hat, a few heads of wheat tucked into the brim. Dressed in a plaid shirt and jeans, with a broad smile that nearly reached his gray sideburns, he looked so much the part of a Montana farmer that he could have been the cover model for a Department of Agriculture outreach publication.

"That guy," Matt said, "is one of the few people in America who is actually serious about building a twenty-first-century economy."

I walked back to my own workstation to do some internet searches of my own. I found out that Bob Quinn was a wheat farmer from Big Sandy, Montana—the same six-hundred-person town that Jon Tester was from. In 1986, Bob had been among the first farmers in the state to go organic—and three years later, he'd served on the national board that advised the US Department of Agriculture in creating standards for the USDA Organic Seal. He'd also started a grain-cleaning plant and flour mill that had been pioneers in premium whole grain, along with the wind farm Matt had shown me on his computer. And Bob was most famous as the entrepreneur behind Kamut wheat, an ancient grain that had gained worldwide popularity for its sweet, nutty flavor and health benefits.

As I clicked through a series of stories about Bob, I found that he was a difficult guy to pigeonhole. He had won a Lifetime of Service Award from the Montana Organic Association, but he had also served on the Wheat Committee of the American Farm Bureau, a mainstream farm organization distrusted by most organic advocates for its vociferous support of feedlots and genetically modified organisms, or GMOs. The US Small Business Administration had named him Small Business Exporter of the Year for Montana in 1995, but most of the stories I found lauded him as a champion of the *local* economy. He had a PhD in plant biochemistry from the University of California, Davis, but he had spent his entire adult life far removed from academia, on a remote farm about seventy miles south of the Canadian border. Most surprising to me, though, was his political affiliation. I had been referred to this eccentric entrepreneur by one of the most politically savvy Democratic staffers I knew, but Bob was identified in multiple news stories as a registered Republican.

I tried to think of a delicate way to ask my boss about our office's relationship with his politically conservative neighbor, not wanting to commit a major faux pas just a few months into my tenure on the Hill. I finally caught a moment with the senator while we were walking down the hallway to greet a group of Montana schoolkids on a field trip. "So, what do you think about Bob Quinn?" I blurted out. "Visionary," Jon responded without hesitating. "This is the guy our founders had in mind when they imagined a democratic nation of enterprising small farmers. We could use a few more people like him up here on the Hill."

"But, umm, isn't he a Republican?" I asked, feeling a little awkward about it. "Oh gosh, maybe," Jon answered nonchalantly, as though we were talking about his neighbor's favorite color or how strong he liked his coffee. "His dad was real active in local Republican politics, and I suspect Bob's voted on the R side a few times himself. Jon added, a twinkle in his eye, "Although, I'm pretty sure he voted for me.

"Look, there's plenty of things we don't agree about," Jon continued, gathering from my puzzled expression that he hadn't quite answered my question. "But the main thing I'm up against here in DC is not Republicans; it's multinational corporations that have a stranglehold on agriculture and energy and don't give a lick about the hardworking Montanans whose livelihoods depend on these industries. Instead of being beholden to these multinationals, we need to build our own economic opportunity, based on renewable resources and good, green jobs that won't go away after the next oil boom. And that's what Bob Quinn is doing."

Three years later, in the summer of 2012, I came back to my hometown of Missoula, Montana. I was now a graduate student working on a dissertation about the roots of the state's booming organic farming sector, which had grown to become one of the largest in the nation. Early in my research, I contacted the foremost scholar on the subject, a University of Montana professor named Neva Hassanein. To my delight, Neva invited me to come over for tea in her backyard.

I showed up on a sunny July afternoon with notebook in hand. A rural sociologist and bastion of progressive organizing in tie-dyed and peace-sign-waving Missoula, Neva was as exuberant as the unruly cascade of curly dark hair that tumbled over her shoulders and down her back. She spoke with great admiration about the diverse farmer-to-farmer groups with whom she had conducted her dissertation research in Wisconsin, including members of a women's network who were reshaping the gender dynamics of their industry. Like her research partners, Neva was committed to making the food system more sustainable and inclusive. Her house was full of canvas farmers market bags.

"I just got back from sabbatical research with Bob Quinn and the Kamut project," Neva beamed, throwing me for a loop. I tried to imagine a conversation between this flamboyantly progressive professor and the man in the cowboy hat whom I'd first seen in the photo Matt had shown me on the internet. I asked Neva what was so special about Bob's work that she'd chosen to spend her sabbatical studying it.

"Most people think Kamut wheat is just a heritage organic grain that's high in selenium," Neva continued, "but it's also a business model for a profoundly different economy. Remember 2008, when the price of conventional grain went through the roof and dozens of farmers ditched their organic certification to sell into the conventional market? The farmers growing for Bob's Kamut project stuck with him—and his buyers negotiated their prices to make it work. He's built this little oasis of trust that is totally the opposite of the race to the bottom going on in corporate America. He has this radical idea that you should value things—people, wheat, land—based on what they're really worth."

A week later, I was on my way to meet the man himself at his farm in Big Sandy. The occasion was the grand opening for Bob's latest venture, The Oil Barn. Neva had explained the concept to me: Bob's plan was to grow safflower, press it into oil, sell it to University of Montana Dining Services for culinary use, and then use the waste oil to fuel his tractor. The whole thing was still in the pilot phase, but Bob was hoping to scale up so that more of his neighbors could grow their own fuel. This grand opening celebration was a big part of that strategy.

I arrived early, but the makeshift parking lot along Bob's driveway was already filling up. A head-turningly diverse crowd streamed in, from TV reporters and politicians in suits to farmers in overalls and college students with piercings and colorfully dyed hair. I saw my old boss, Senator Tester, standing near a podium that had been set up under an old box elder tree in Bob's backyard. Someone tapped the microphone and we gathered around a few rows of white folding chairs.

I knew Bob the moment I saw him. He was wearing the same cowboy hat he'd had on in the photo from the wind farm's grand opening, with those heads of ancient wheat in the brim. "In the days of the American Revolution," he began, "every village had a liberty tree where people would get together to talk about freedom and how they were going to achieve it." The crowd silenced their conversations and leaned in.

"And today we're gathered under this box elder," Bob continued, gesturing to the verdant tree next to him, "to talk about freedom from being beholden to others for our energy."

Several dozen heads nodded in unison, a concert of ball caps, cowboy hats, carefully slicked-back hairdos, and a few longhairs. Now I understood what Matt, Jon, and Neva had been trying to tell me. Bob was a true champion for the public good. And the public—the whole motley lot of us—could see that he was in earnest. The usual categories didn't seem to matter.

Over the next five years, Bob and I bumped into each other more and more often. I continued my research on Montana sustainable agriculture, and Bob's name came up frequently during my interviews. Once I finished my PhD, published a book, and began teaching at Stanford University, Bob and I found ourselves at the same organic agriculture conferences, delivering similar messages about the link between healthy soil, healthy food, and a healthy rural economy. One summer day in 2017, we ran across each other at a Montana Organic Association farm tour, hosted by a grass-fed beef operation about an hour's drive north of Bob's place. There were several stops on the all-day tour, accessible only by four-wheel-drive pickup trucks that could navigate ranch roads. My partner and I had driven to the tour in a rental sedan, so we hitched a ride in Bob's pickup.

As we climbed out of the truck to look at a brilliant yellow pasture of soil-building sweet clover, Bob made a little side comment. "So, Liz, you know I've been thinking about writing a book," he said. "I've been told I should get a ghostwriter, but I'd rather have more of an equal partner in the project, someone who could contribute their own knowledge and ideas."

In the next five seconds, I finally had to confront the question myself. The question I'd asked Jon. The question I'd wanted to ask Neva. Were the things Bob and I had in common more important than our differences?

"Bob, I think you should do that book," I said. "And I want to help you write it."

What you now hold in your hands is the story of an unsung hero—a small-town farmer who is rebuilding his rural community, one opportunity at a time. By creating a market for organic, whole grain ancient wheat, he's helped more than a hundred other farmers convert to more environmentally friendly and economically stable practices. By launching a wind farm and a biofuel project, he's pushed Montana toward renewable energy, which has accounted for the majority of the state's new energy capacity since Bob got involved fifteen years ago.[1] All the while, he's insisted that we can't keep building an economy based on cheapness: cheap fuel, cheap food, cheap labor. Ultimately, that kind of economy means we're undervaluing ourselves and our neighbors. It means diabetes and poverty, water pollution and bankruptcy. Instead, we need to build an economy based on honest value. Jobs. Community.

Health. Sustainability. In a little corner of Montana, Bob has been working to create that kind of economy, and he's an inspiration to the growing circle of people who've now entered his orbit from all across the political spectrum.

Here, in his own words, is Bob's hopeful vision for a more prosperous future, along with the story of how he got to where he is today. I've helped with some of the research and writing, mostly to draw out the larger context and significance of the events in the book. But I'm leaving my first-person voice aside from here on because I want you to get to know this green economy cowboy for yourself, not secondhand from me. In the warm, humorous, straight-shooting manner in which only Bob can render his experience, I think you'll find a good deal of practical wisdom. And, if I may toot his horn a bit, a genuine American hero.

Food on the Cheap

I remember the day I stopped trying to grow food on the cheap.

Born into a family wheat and cattle operation in Montana during the baby boom, I'd grown up accepting the conventional wisdom about American farmers: that our job was to feed the world, and that to do so, we needed to produce the highest possible yields by any means necessary. Over the course of my lifetime, Americans cut in half the percentage of their income they spent on food.[1] The number of Americans working in agriculture dwindled too: from nearly 6.7 million in 1947, the year I was born, to just 2 million today.[2] These trends were hailed as signs of progress.

In 1971, as a freshly minted college graduate, I ventured into the heart of that progress: the University of California, Davis, arguably the top agricultural school in the country. Our professors wanted us graduate students to see the innovative practices of modern farming firsthand, so they took us on a number of field trips. We visited massive orange groves in Southern California, vegetable operations on the Central Coast, and timber operations in the mountains. But the trip I remember most vividly was our outing to a peach farm in California's

1

Central Valley, one of the most productive farming regions in the world.

En route to the farm, I found myself daydreaming about the sweet aroma of ripe peaches, the sticky satisfaction of their juicy flesh. Of course, my parents couldn't grow peaches in chilly north central Montana, so in my childhood they had been a rare treat. I remember those special occasion peaches arriving at our local grocery store, meticulously wrapped in tissue paper and placed in paper cups, which were carefully nestled in wooden crates. We would take them home and set them out on the counter for a few days, where they would ripen to sweet, succulent perfection. When I moved to Davis for graduate school, I was delighted to discover a small peach farm just down the road, near Woodland. My wife and I were on a limited graduate student budget with a couple babies in the house already, so we asked the farmer if we could buy from him in bulk and can our own winter fruit supply. "Well, will you be canning today, tomorrow, or in a few days?" the farmer asked. When we answered "Today," the farmer pointed us to a stack of boxes teeming with dead-ripe fruit right off the tree. It took all the discipline we could muster to actually can all those peaches and not just start scarfing them down on the spot. This was the image I had in my mind as I left for the field trip to the Central Valley peach farm, which was serendipitously scheduled at harvesttime.

When my fellow students and I arrived at the farm, I stepped off the bus into a sea of peach trees, stretching as far as the eye could see. I took a deep breath, expecting to be overwhelmed by the scent of ripe peaches. But strangely enough, I couldn't smell them.

That's when I noticed my professor and the peach grower, standing to the side of the crowd and laughing. They were talking about a petroleum-based product the professor had developed that the grower was spraying on his peaches. The spray stimulated the skin of the peaches to change color so they *looked* ripe, even though they were still green as grass and not fit to eat. These rock-hard peaches could then be shipped across the country in bulk, without the expense of careful packaging to prevent bruising. The grower and the professor were both in a position to profit, and yet these peaches could also be sold more cheaply in grocery stores, where they would, hopefully, ripen up enough to be palatable.

As a PhD student in plant biochemistry, I knew unripe peaches didn't have the same nutritional profile as ripe ones. I suspected this petroleum-based spray wasn't good for the environment, and I wondered what residues might be left on the fruit. Something was wrong with this kind of agriculture and, for that matter, with the kind of economy that drove it. I stayed at Davis to finish my PhD, but the more I saw of this so-called modern agriculture, the more concerned I became. In 1978, I returned home to take over my parents' Montana wheat farm, determined to do things differently. If I could.

The past fifty years of American history can be summed up in three remarkably similar graphs of three ostensibly different things. One shows a steady rise in the percentage of the US population with diagnosed diabetes, from less than 1 percent in 1958 to nearly 10 percent today.[3] Another shows a very similar trend line in the average carbon dioxide concentration at the Mauna Loa Observatory in Hawaii—this is the famous Keeling Curve, which first sounded the alarm on climate change. The third graph shows the number of Americans reliant on food stamps, which has risen from just over 10 million in 1972 to more than 45 million today.[4] The correlation in these trends is no accident—they are all symptomatic of a system of producing and consuming goods, particularly food, that has gone badly awry. Unless we begin to change this system, these statistics will continue to rise, with disastrous consequences for our health, our livelihoods, and our planet.

The mistake we've made these past fifty years? As a nation, we've simply become too cheap, particularly when it comes to food. Achieving this extraordinary cheapness has meant continually extracting value out of the entire supply chain that leads to our suppers—from the farms and rural communities where our food is grown, to the processing facilities and fast-food restaurants where underpaid workers scramble to churn out meals cheaper and faster, to the dinner table, where we encounter increasingly calorie-rich and nutrient-poor fare. As this value is extracted from our communities, much of it is being transformed into something that meets no clear human need: increased profits for the already bloated multinational corporations that have cornered the market on food processing, retail, and agricultural chemicals.

This is a book about how to add that value back where it belongs, not only to the end product—our food—but to the entire food system. As an entrepreneur and scientist working in the midst of rural American poverty, I have seen firsthand how putting food and other fundamental goods like energy at the center of a value-added economy can foster health, economic opportunity, and ecological regeneration, particularly in some of our country's poorest communities. The truth is, cheap stuff isn't really cheap—the bill just comes due somewhere downstream or down the line. Likewise, adding value isn't expensive—it's actually a remarkably efficient way to reduce the soaring costs of health care, poverty, and environmental degradation, all of which are putting a strain on our national budget. Adding value to our food means we can regenerate land instead of destroying it. We can revitalize rural communities instead of giving up on them. We can heal people instead of making them sick.

When I returned to my family's farm, I realized that the primary crop we grew—wheat—was trying to tell us something. Believed to be among the first plants domesticated by humans some ten thousand years ago, this prolific grass soon became the staff of life for ancient civilizations from Babylonia to Persia to Han China to Rome.[5] Up until the past century or so, wheat—in the form of bread—made up the bulk of the diet for most Europeans,[6] and as recently as the 1930s and 1940s, Americans obtained more of their calories from bread than from any other food.[7] Nutrient dense and suited to a variety of growing conditions, wheat remains the most widely planted crop today, accounting for one-fifth of the calories in the human diet.[8] But 15 to 20 percent of Americans say they can no longer comfortably eat it.

As an increasing number of my friends and neighbors came down with symptoms of "gluten sensitivity," I read everything I could get my hands on to try to understand what might be wrong with our wheat. At first, there wasn't much to read: early on, these wheat-sensitive people were waved off as hypochondriacs. But in the past ten years, there has been a flood of diet books, cookbooks, and gluten-free manifestos, all offering explanations and solutions for individuals who have trouble digesting wheat products. These books have offered relief for millions of suffering people and validated their experience with at least some degree of sound science about the interaction between the wheat they are eating and their digestive systems. I think these gluten-free guidebooks are right to condemn most of the wheat in the contemporary American diet as lacking in nutrition and ill-suited to our bodies' needs. And yet, none of these books have answered the burning question nagging at me: if we've been eating wheat for ten thousand years, why has it suddenly started giving us trouble?

To me, there is something almost sacred about growing wheat. Nearly every spring of my life, I have held in my hands a seed passed down over five hundred generations, a seed that has nourished my fellow humans for some ten millennia. Holding that wheat seed in my hands, I feel connected to the billions of my human brothers and sisters who have turned to this same grain to break bread with one another: to nourish, to celebrate, to earn an honest living. So much of what is meaningful in human life is there in that grain. I struggle to fully comprehend the value of this gift.

There is another way to think about the value of this wheat, however. The Nasdaq Stock Market lists the price every day, by the bushel. For example, on September 13, 2017, as we were drafting this chapter, the price of wheat was $4.20 per bushel—about a penny per serving.

If a penny per serving sounds like a bargain, it is. Sort of. To produce wheat this cheaply, you need to grow a lot of it as inexpensively as possible. Buyers constantly attempt to drive down prices, to the point that farmers can barely eke out a living. Farmers, in turn, scramble to maximize production in order to survive on such small margins. In a desperate attempt to increase yields, they've turned to herbicides like glyphosate, now classified by the International Agency for Research on Cancer as a probable human carcinogen.[9] And to boost both yields and protein premiums, they apply copious amounts of synthetic nitrogen fertilizer—typically beyond what the plants can use. The excess nitrogen acidifies our soils, so they are less productive[10]—then runs off into the watershed, where it can lead to contaminated drinking water and hypoxic "dead zones" that suffocate the life in our lakes and coastal areas.[11]

Meanwhile, the nutritious wheat varieties passed down over five hundred generations have become a rarity. In place of this rich diversity of wheat, painstakingly selected and adapted to different growing regions over thousands of years, contemporary plant breeders have substituted a handful of recently developed varieties. These new varieties are bred primarily for high yield and loaf volume, which increases the number of loaves of bread industrial processors can squeeze out of each bag of flour by pumping as much air into the dough as quickly as possible. When raised under ideal growing conditions, with plentiful supplies of fertilizer, pesticides, and water, today's wheat varieties do yield much more grain than the varieties planted by our forebears. But the environmental consequences of such chemically intensive agriculture are beginning to add up, and all this cheap modern grain is antagonizing people's digestive systems and devastating rural America.

As a young boy growing up in one of the country's premier wheat-producing regions, I began to notice these changes as they transformed my family's Montana farm. As a young man taking the reins of that farm in the early 1980s, I started asking myself the same question I'd asked in that peach orchard in California: are we going in the wrong direction?

I was also troubled by the realization that the farm's finances had very little to do with the quality of our work. In those days, we got paid in two ways. The federal government mailed us a subsidy check based on the number of acres of wheat we planted every year and our proven yield. Then, once we had harvested the crop and hauled it to our local grain elevator, we were paid a per-bushel price that fluctuated wildly based on global market dynamics far removed from the farm. Neither method of compensation rewarded us for doing the things that really mattered: growing high-quality food and responsibly stewarding our land. Instead, both the government and the grain buyers sized up our wheat as they would any other standardized, industrial product. Wheat was not referred to as food. It was a commodity. All that counted, in the words of US Secretary of Agriculture Earl Butz, was that we planted every acre of our farm, "fencerow to fencerow," and hauled off as many bushels of grain as possible. In order to maximize production, farmers had to rely on high inputs of fertilizers and pesticides instead of regenerating their soils to sustain the long-term health of the farm. This chemical dependence undermined their own long-term profitability, along with their communities, the environment, and public health.

Meanwhile, I eventually learned, the people making real money on wheat weren't farmers but the companies selling us all those chemical inputs—and the Wall Street firms that ultimately came to control 40 percent of wheat futures.[12] I imagined groups of men in three-piece suits exchanging papers in the comfort of air-conditioned offices while they discussed a crop they'd probably never even seen and would not recognize if they'd been standing in a field of it. Through clever buying and selling strategies, they were able to make far more money than I could make out in the hot sun growing wheat in the first place.

If farmers were shafted by such a system, I began to realize, eaters were not much better off. On the supermarket shelves of their local grocery stores, they had little choice outside of standardized commodity wheat, crushed between colossal steel rollers to strip it of its nutrient-dense bran and germ. Processors did their best to package this white flour into creative forms, giving the appearance of an abundance of culinary options: vitamin-fortified white bread, fiber-added breakfast cereal, omega 3–enriched energy bars—all packed with sugar and a host of unpronounceable ingredients meant to increase shelf life and make the stuff taste like food. The processors even had the audacity to call such concoctions "value-added products."

To me, this definition of "value added" is completely backward. Many things have been added to our commodity wheat, but value is not one of them. We would never have needed nutrient fortification in the first place if we hadn't removed so many nutrients in the course of industrial breeding, production, and processing. When we look at the *net* movement of value in the commodity system, it's pretty clear that it has been moving steadily *away* from our food. What we have now is essentially *value-subtracted* wheat. Not only has much of the embedded value been literally stripped away—no bran, no germ, no soil health, often no net profit to the farmer—the ability to even assess value in such terms has been removed too. The purveyors of value-subtracted products deliberately conceal the nature of their production and processing: as the saying goes, no one wants to know how the sausage is made.

In contemporary American society, we see many such value-subtracted products. Commodity wheat, corn, and soy, aggressively refined and transformed into soda and burgers and cookies, greet you in nearly every aisle of the supermarket. The car you probably drove to get there runs on value-subtracted energy: commodity petroleum. The clothes you're wearing? Value-subtracted fiber: commodity cotton, or perhaps a blend of synthetics.

The supposed benefit of all these value-subtracted products is that they are cheap and abundant. But cheap for whom and abundant at what cost? The price paid at the cash register is deceptive. The real tab starts to add up when you account for the costs of the chronic diseases related to all our cheap foods. The bill gets even steeper when you consider the cost to struggling farmers forced to sell their land and move on, and to the rural communities that lose their schools and hospitals as their population empties out. Then there are all the other poorly paid people along the supply chain: fast-food workers, processing plant workers, grocery store clerks. Plus the environmental damage, from the New Jersey–size dead zone our fertilizer runoff has created in the Gulf of Mexico to the hundreds of megatons of carbon dioxide we add to the atmosphere every year to manufacture those fertilizers.[13] When you start adding up all the costs of cheap food, value subtraction begins to look quite expensive. We're not really saving money. We're just sticking ourselves and our kids with a hefty tab to pay down the road. And meanwhile, we're pouring our local resources into the pockets of a few wealthy multinationals who make the big money in the food system, absorbing their costs in the form of poor health, pollution, poverty, and the billions of taxpayer dollars spent trying to fix these problems.

What about low-income folks on tight budgets, you might ask—don't they need to economize? How can they afford to pay more for their groceries? Low-income earners, however, are perhaps the most disadvantaged by the cheap food system—many are low income because they work poorly paid jobs in the food sector, and many more bear an outsize share of the environmental and health burdens of our industrial food system.[14] Meanwhile, many of the people purchasing cheap food do so despite the fact that they have income to spare: a pair of economists recently analyzed Americans' fast-food purchases and found the frequency strikingly similar for people of all income levels.[15]

How did twenty-first-century Americans arrive at the most shortsighted notion of value in the history of the world? I think the heart of the problem is our commodity mentality, the disconnect that comes from buying and selling an anonymous, standardized product with little information about where it came from or where it is going. The commodity mentality makes farmers forget that they are growing food. It makes eaters forget that what they are eating originated on a farm. Both parties see only the up-front price, which gives the mistaken impression that they are adversaries: consumers demanding lower prices versus producers demanding higher ones. When we broaden our view from this focus on price to a more comprehensive accounting of value, however, we see a very different picture.

"Value," according to *Merriam-Webster*, means more than just price. It also means "a fair return" for goods or services. It's not just about what people will pay for something but what that something brings to the table in "worth, utility, or importance." And, critically, *Merriam-Webster*'s definition of value also accounts for "intrinsically" worthy or important things: what we commonly refer to as our values.

What I've come to understand in the course of my four decades in business is that this more comprehensive form of value—what we really ought to be building—is not necessarily adversarial. When we begin reconnecting the dots between our soils and our suppers, we see that a healthy food system benefits everybody—the farmer who wants to maintain productive fields, the eater who wants a nutritious meal, the neighbor downstream who wants clean drinking water. The value of our most fundamental goods, like food and energy, connects everyone on the planet—producer and consumer alike—to the reality that we get what we pay for.

I didn't set out to condemn the cheap food economy or the commodity system—or even call them into question. Forty years ago, I was just a kid coming back to my parents' wheat and cattle ranch, looking to support the family business and earn enough additional income to provide for my own growing family. But like many other people across America, I've found this seemingly simple objective—to earn an honest living—quite a bit more complex than I expected. As I've learned over the course of five business ventures and a lifetime of fighting to keep my small town alive, business as usual is not a viable option. The only way forward is a paradigm shift—toward a fuller notion of value that puts the long-term well-being of people, communities, and land before the short-term goal of solely maximizing profit and efficiencies. In other words, we need to start focusing a lot more on quality rather than just quantity.

The premise of this book is that economics is not just about what happens in faraway boardrooms or on the floor of the stock market. The real measures of economic health are in the fundamental goods that not only make our lives possible but also make them worth living: thriving communities, meaningful work, healthy land. At the center of this fundamental economy are our staple foods, our daily bread. If we hope to recover honest value in American society, we must redeem the original commodity, wheat.

This is the deeper promise behind the many small steps I've taken to add value to my business as a wheat farmer. When a few other processors and I started milling our grain whole, in the 1980s, we wanted to bring back the nutritional value that had been refined away for the past century. When I converted my farm to organic, at about the same time, I wanted to bring back the life in my soil, to support more profitable crops and a healthier environment. And when I began rediscovering heirloom grains—the seeds our ancestors planted—I realized just how much taste and nutrition we'd sacrificed in the rush to breed high-yielding varieties.

But as I kept looking to add fundamental value to my business, it soon became evident that this was not just about wheat. As we built markets for heirloom, organic whole grain, local mills and bakeries started popping up again. After generations of outmigration, young people began returning to rural communities, starting small enterprises, and raising families. My hometown of Big Sandy, once in danger of becoming an empty spot on the map, started to feel like a *place* again.

This budding revival of wheat—back to its former status as the staff of life—has given me hope, not just for this crop but for the future of our society and our planet. Looking out over my fields, I see that we may finally be moving away from a commodity mentality in favor of products that explicitly assign value to soil quality, rural livelihoods, climate stability, and human health. Doctors are now venturing out into farm fields, declaring that responsible, chemical-free agriculture is at the root of improving public health.[16]

This is also happening with other crops besides wheat. Americans now buy $50 billion worth of organic food every year—over 5 percent of total US food sales.[17] The US market for grass-fed beef is growing at 100 percent per year.[18] And nearly half the money spent on coffee in the United States goes to specialty varieties distinguished by quality, sustainability, or the share of the profit earned by the farmer.[19]

As farmers and artisans find ways to distinguish high-quality food from cheap commodities, I often hear these higher-quality products referred to as "value added." This, of course, is the term processors adopted in the early twentieth century to make it sound as if white flour fortified with vitamins was better than whole wheat flour, which is naturally nutrient dense. A better term for these fortified processed foods, I think, would be "value subtracted" because from a net value perspective, the consumer is losing. Meanwhile, foods that offer real value—whole foods that haven't been stripped of their most nutritious elements—should be differentiated in another way. I think it would be more accurate to refer to ecologically raised whole foods as "value not subtracted," but that doesn't have quite the same ring to it as "value added," and the commodity processors would probably sue us for food libel. I suppose from the standpoint of a predominantly industrial food system, we are indeed adding value, but let's be reasonable about it: we're adding it back.

Whatever you call these value-not-subtracted products, they tend to be waved off as charming stories for the human interest page. Filler for gift baskets. Luxuries for foodies. Painted into the corner of "niche markets," they are conceived as a pretty little sideshow to the flood of cheap commodities that we are told is the backbone of the agricultural economy and the safeguard of global food security.

And yet, the consequences of value subtraction are everywhere screaming for acknowledgment: Decimation of rural communities. Epidemics of diet-related chronic disease. A planet besieged by climate turmoil, one-third of which can be attributed to food and agriculture. Water supplies contaminated and overtaxed. One-fifth of the world's farmland degraded. Pollinators in decline. As one panel of global authorities put it, the commodity food, fiber, and energy system is "an existential threat to itself"[20]—and thus to all of us.

Meanwhile, the value-not-subtracted sector is beginning to revitalize our food system and what is left of our rural communities—helping family farms survive, returning soil health to millions of acres of certified organic farmland, and innovating some of the most promising greenhouse gas drawdown solutions on the planet. In the face of widespread digestive problems and bleak statistics about chronic disease, this value-not-subtracted food also offers something of great importance to eaters: a lifeline of nutrition. Many of these eaters—as well as many of the institutions that serve them—have begun to rethink the notion that cheap food is a bargain. Instead of demanding low prices, they are demanding high value—which means building genuine partnerships with producers rather than simply asking them to grow food in whatever way minimizes the share of the cost that is paid at the point of sale.

It's sort of like the signs you sometimes see on a busy residential street that encourage motorists to "drive like your kids live here." We need to eat like our kids live here. After all, our food comes from the same planet, the same communities we are passing on to our children. This becomes vividly clear when you farm or grow a garden. That compost you added last year leaves your soil moist and spongy. The spot where you plowed too early, when the ground was still wet, is compacted and hard to seed. From here, it's not too hard to understand that everything we eat comes from a place to which we are connected, a place with which our fates are intertwined. We don't need to grow all our own food, or source all of it locally—although I think we should do far more of both of these things than most of us do in today's United States. But we should *value* our food, and everything it takes to get it to our plates, as though it were homegrown. Because, in a sense, it is.

Over the course of the past forty years, I've learned a series of vivid lessons about the far-reaching consequences of economics as usual and the potential of rekindling a more honest, direct relationship with our everyday necessities. This journey has taken me to Egyptian wheat fields, Italian pasta factories, Russian seed vaults, and the headquarters of the US Department of Agriculture in Washington, DC. It's forced me to rethink the way I raise plants, the way I do business, and what it means to be successful. But it all started with a seemingly simple objective: to earn a viable living on my family farm.

CHAPTER 1:

Roots and Growth

When I was a sophomore at Big Sandy High School, we started a new club: speech and debate. I liked it better than any other extracurricular activity because it was easy to make friends with people from all over the state. In sports, you shook hands with the other team after the game, but you didn't really mix with them much—the objective was to beat them. Speech was different. We talked to each other. Sometimes I learned surprising things.

To me, the 950-person town of Big Sandy, Montana, was a minor metropolis. Movie theater, swimming pool, skating rink—when I got to go to town, which was about a fifteen-mile drive from my family's farm, I thought we had an amazing number of things to do. But my friends who lived right in the thick of it would say, "Oh, this is just a hole; there's nothing to do here." On and on about how bored they were. Geez, I thought, you should live out in the country by yourself and see how magical it is to have a movie theater right down Main Street.

When I started to do speech and debate, I met kids from a larger town thirty-five miles northeast of Big Sandy that my folks took me to sometimes on special occasions: Havre. In Havre, they had *three* movie theaters. They even had an outdoor theater, or a drive-in, as we called it, and an A&W stand where they served root beer in frozen mugs. When the A&W soda jerks poured the root beer into the mug, it would freeze a little bit around the rim, so you'd have these ice crystals at the top of the glass. That cost a nickel, for the medium size. On a very special occasion, I sometimes got a root beer float, which was twenty-five cents. I would look forward to that for months. But when I got acquainted with a guy from Havre who did speech and debate, he said, "Oh, this is just a hole; there's nothing to do here." Curious, I thought, that's just what my friends from Big Sandy said.

Then I started to meet kids from Great Falls. Now, this was the big time. In Montana, the first number on your license plate indicates what county you're from, and it's in approximate order of the population size as of the 1930 census. Great Falls was number two, just behind Butte. They had the state fair, all kinds of stores and things to do. They had swimming pools *indoors*. And yet, the Great Falls kids said the same thing: "This is just a hole." They had their eyes on the really big cities out of state.

At that point, I think it dawned on me: You can always look for someplace bigger and better. Or you can make the most of where you are.

The Big Sandy of my childhood was a hub of activity. We had a post office, two hotels, a drugstore, a jeweler, two secondhand stores, a lumberyard, a bank, three grocery stores, two restaurants, a clothing store, a couple of gas stations, a Chevy dealership, a public library, a dry cleaner, a law office, an accounting firm, an agricultural equipment dealer, and two hardware stores. In addition to the swimming pool in the summer and the skating rink in the winter, we had a bowling alley and a combination pool hall and soda fountain where you could buy a hamburger and a Coke for forty-five cents. We had five grain elevators, five bars, and five churches, so we thought we were pretty balanced.

We held country dances in the schoolhouse that would start at eight or nine and go all night. Polkas, waltzes, schottisches, square dances—I would practice out behind the barn until I had the steps down. We would eat a midnight supper and then keep dancing until two or three in the morning, sometimes later. In the summertime, it would be getting light when we went home.

The farm I grew up on was a half hour's drive southeast of town, surrounded by windswept prairie. From my front porch, I could see for miles around. Sixty miles to the south were the Judith Mountains, and on a clear day I could even see the taller range beyond them, the Little Belts. Eighty miles northwest, along the Canadian border, were the Sweet Grass Hills. And just a few miles away, the Bear Paw Mountains rose up to the northeast in a jagged sweep of indigo. My grandfather had started farming the place in 1920, and my dad had taken over in 1948, a year after I was born. It was a midsize family operation for those days: 2,400 acres, half wheat, half cattle.

My grandfather and my dad knew all of their cows individually, even though there were nearly fifty. They could say, "That cow over there, she's the one that has the small calves." "She's ornery" or "She's docile"; "She's the leader" or "She's the follower."

We knew all our neighbors too. One of our closest neighbors had the binder that we would borrow every year to cut our oats for our cattle's winter feed. One of my very first jobs on the farm was to ride that binder, which my dad pulled behind our tractor. It was an amazing machine: it not only cut the oats but also tied them into foot-thick bundles, which it dumped out one by one on a little platform. My task, as soon as I was big enough to push and pull the appropriate lever, was to dump these bundles onto the field once the platform filled up, so more bundles could be collected. Once I got a little older, I graduated to the burlier job of walking through the field after the binder went through and stacking the oat bundles against one another

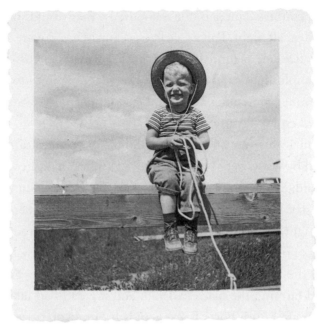

ON THE CORRAL FENCE WITH MY FIRST COWBOY HAT AND ROPE,
KEEPING AN EYE ON THE COWS AT QUINN FARM & RANCH.
(Photo by John Miller)

so they would dry properly. In the early fall, when I was back in school, my dad would come back for the dried bundles, pitch them into a wagon, and haul them back to the hammer mill next to the barn. The hammer mill chopped the oats into little two- or three-inch pieces and blew them into the feed shed, where our cows enjoyed them throughout the winter.

Hauling our oat bundles into the barn every fall took my dad the better part of a week, so he was eager to purchase a machine that could chop the oats right in the field, eliminating an awful lot of binding and gathering of bundles. But upgrading our oat harvest meant purchasing a whole fleet of additional machinery: a swather, which would cut the oat plants down and lay them in windrows; a chopper, which would pick up the windrows and chop them; a customized truck, into which the chopper would blow the shredded oats; and a blower, which would neatly usher this load of feed straight from our truck to our barn. It was a big investment, so we partnered with the same neighbors and bought one swather, chopper, and blower to share. We each outfitted a truck for the job, but we lent them to one another during harvest time so that one truck could gather oats while the other loaded them into the blower. Neighbors often helped each other with tasks like these, just as we did when it came time to brand cattle or raise a new building. I tagged along with my dad on countless cement-pouring projects for new barns and homes around the neighborhood.

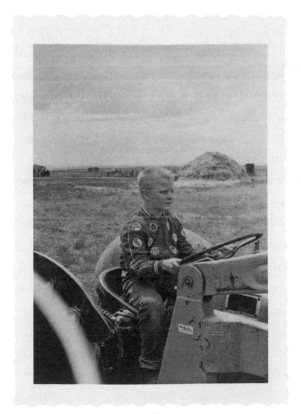

READY TO HEAD TO THE FIELD ON MY FIRST TRACTOR, AGE TEN.
(Photo courtesy of Bob Quinn)

In August, though, all other activity stopped for the wheat harvest. Part of the Golden Triangle region of north central Montana, the Big Sandy area was known for its production of high-protein wheat, which flowed out of the fields in late summer like a river of gold. There were five grain elevators in town to haul our crops to. Three were owned by a large out-of-state corporation. One was run by the local chapter of the Farmers Union, a national farm advocacy group known for organizing producer cooperatives. The fifth, Big Sandy Grain Company, had recently been established by another group of local farmers, many of whom were part of a competing farm advocacy organization, the Farm Bureau.

Looking back all these years later, I realize these two local elevators had pretty similar business models. Local farmers shared in the costs and the proceeds. Decisions were made locally too, according to farmers' best interests. The Farmers Union also had some associated services and a farm supply store, so that was unique, and Big Sandy Grain Company was the first to add a bulk fertilizer plant and a roller mill to roll grain in the winter for feeding cattle. But otherwise, the two rival elevators bore a strong resemblance to each other. At the core of each operation was the same basic principle: keep the money in the local community and negotiate for better prices as a group, rather than taking products to market as individual farmers and getting jerked around by the big grain corporations.

But had I suggested at the time that my dad haul his grain to the Farmers Union elevator, that would have been like telling a Red Sox fan to go cheer for the Yankees. Farmers Union and Farm Bureau were different crowds, and since we were in the Farm Bureau camp, we hauled to Big Sandy Grain Company. The two elevators were on opposite sides of Main Street, and everybody knew who was on which side.

My father, who was a shareholder in Big Sandy Grain Company, was very careful not to call it a "co-op" because that word was associated with the Farmers Union. It was sort of like a dirty word in our crowd, a word that indicated you weren't focused enough on the viability of your business. But of course the Farmers Union elevator had to be viable to stay in business—and in many ways our elevator was replicating their focus on mutual benefit. Some things have improved in farm country since I was a kid, and I think one of them is that Farm Bureau members and Farmers Union members actually talk to each other now and work together. Unfortunately, it wasn't until get-big-or-get-out farm policy had dramatically depopulated rural America—drastically reducing the ranks of both farm organizations—that their members began to recognize that they had more in common than they had to fight about.

Owning our own grain elevators was a step in the right direction for both Farmers Union families and Farm Bureau families like mine, but it still didn't make us masters of our own destiny. Despite the sense of independence we had in our day-to-day lives, we were all selling most of the grain from our local elevators into the global commodity food system—which meant that many aspects of our operations were effectively out of our hands. One of those out-of-our-hands matters that particularly frustrated Big Sandy farmers like my dad was the fact that in order to get our product to market, we had to put our grain on the Great Northern Railway, one of the biggest monopolies in the history of the American West.[1] The behemoth railroad was a constant source of consternation, widely suspected of jacking up prices and resented for making so much profit while its captive shippers—growers—struggled to make ends meet. To add insult to injury, the railroad didn't always send enough cars at harvesttime. Inevitably, the elevators alongside the tracks would get so full that they couldn't accept any more loads. Plugged, we called it. For our neighbors without sufficient grain storage on their own farms, this meant that in years of plentiful harvests they had to dump part of their grain on the ground and pick it up later—a costly and risky proposition.

My father made sure that he had enough steel bins to store everything we grew, so we didn't have to haul it in at harvest if the railcars weren't there. He was very big on backup plans and not putting all his eggs in one basket. In the 1960s, government and economic "experts" were starting to put a lot of pressure on farmers to specialize in one thing or another and maximize their profits. Farm policy reflected these recommendations, incentivizing monoculture. My dad didn't buy it. He liked to keep half the farm in cattle and half in grain, and if he had a bad year with one enterprise, he could usually make it up with the other.

Another thing Dad really believed in was community activities. In between farm chores, he and my mother drove all over the state attending various meetings—he in his Stetson hat, she in her beaver coat and pearls. While Mom took her turn in the lead with the PTA and Sunday school, Dad was a charter member of Big Sandy's chapter of Rotary Club, an international organization of civically oriented businesspeople that spearheaded the building of our local swimming pool and the new hospital. He was a proud member of the American Legion, like his father before him, and he joined up with the Masonic Order and the Shriners too. He never ran for public office—other than the local school board, which he sat on for fifteen years—but he was quite enthusiastic about politics, and my sister Debby and I were expected to participate. I'll never forget the Halloween night in 1964 when we walked around town with "cookies for Goldwater," encouraging people to vote in the upcoming election. Debby and I went up to this one house and knocked on the door. We waited. Finally, an old guy answered, sizing us up. "How's a Democrat with false teeth supposed to eat a Republican cookie?" he barked.

Although Dad didn't become a politician, he did eventually become president of the Montana Farm Bureau and served on the organization's national board of directors. He had earned a reputation as a forward-thinking, innovative producer, having won the title of Montana's Outstanding Young Farmer in 1955. Always on the lookout for new ways to do things better, he was one of the first in our area to start experimenting with chemical fertilizers.

At the time, most of our neighbors thought fertilizers were a waste of money. But soon, it seemed like everybody was using them: US fertilizer application doubled over the course of the 1940s, then nearly doubled again between 1950 and 1970.[2] The ground was beginning to wear out from decades of mining the fertility of the soil, and this was the first serious attempt to put something back. Looking back, I'm convinced it wasn't the right way, but it was the correct principle: add something back to replace what has been removed.

Chemical fertilizers may have been a bit of a tough sell, but herbicides were adopted immediately. They were like a wonder drug. In those days, people practiced very limited crop rotation, and their planting sequences were not nearly complex enough to keep the soil healthy and break up cycles of pests and disease. So the weeds kept getting worse and worse until 2,4-D came along and totally knocked them out in one pass.

I don't remember anybody raising concerns that herbicides might be bad for us. People would spray in open-air tractors with the wind blowing the chemicals back in their face. But I never really liked them much. I could see drift damage curling up the leaves of the ash trees in our shelterbelts. And the worst part was what they did to my garden.

Contrary to the fantasy version of rural life, we didn't live entirely off the fat of the land, the way my grandparents had. My mother bought "air bread" from town—the same fluffy white stuff nearly everybody had in the 1950s—rather than making her own, and she wasn't big on growing vegetables. But my great-aunt who lived in Big Sandy had more of a green thumb. She baked her own bread—which of course we thought had too hard a crust and a weirdly grainy flavor (probably because it actually tasted like grain). And she gardened.

When I was still in grade school my great-aunt got me a subscription to Rodale's *Organic Gardening* magazine, and she and my grandfather helped me grow a small garden. I loved it. I planted all sorts of things: carrots, tomatoes, peas, beets, beans, chard, radishes, sweet corn. Being very Irish, my grandfather insisted I plant potatoes on Good Friday, and my fall harvest included buttercup squash and pumpkins for Halloween.

Showing up at the front door of our house with freshly picked ears of corn for my mother or a Halloween pumpkin for my grandmother filled me with a distinct kind of pride, notably different from the satisfaction I got out of accomplishing other kinds of everyday tasks and chores. Planting a seed, nurturing it, watching it grow, harvesting its bounty, and sharing it with someone I loved made me feel like I was making a real contribution of my own, not just following somebody else's instructions. Inspired, I started making ice cream from the fresh milk and cream I got from our milk cow, then bringing it to school for special class events. I wasn't very good with art or mechanical things, and I didn't have the money to buy presents for my friends. And yet, when I came to school with that ice cream, I was as big a hero as the football quarterback. Meanwhile, I continued to do the same thing with my garden: grow things and give them away.

But then my father would come back to the house after spraying herbicide on our grain crop, and he would walk by my little vegetable plot with his coveralls on. Mom made him take them off before he went into the house, but he still had them on when he walked by the garden. My plants that were next to the sidewalk withered. They just curled up and died.

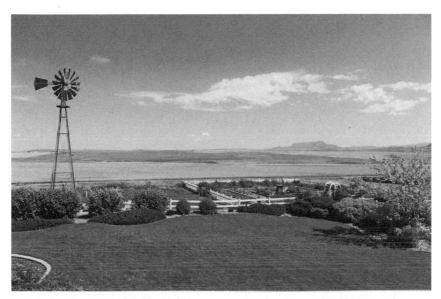

QUINN FARM & RANCH, WITH MY CURRENT GARDEN IN THE FOREGROUND
AND THE BEAR PAW MOUNTAINS IN THE DISTANCE.
(Photo by Hilary Page)

The decade after World War II was a good time to be an American farmer. The weather was kind, the rains were sufficient, and the federal farm programs established in response to the Great Depression of the 1930s helped ensure that grain prices were adequate to compensate growers for their labor. The Marshall Plan sent American grain to war-ravaged Europe, meaning US farmers had a guaranteed market.[3] Agricultural policies, by and large, were designed to support rural communities rather than just the products that flowed out of them.

In truth, we were not really a nation of farmers anymore: in 1950, farm residents accounted for just 15.3 percent of the total US population. But just a generation earlier, that figure had been as high as one-quarter; two generations earlier it had been as high as one-third.[4] Consequently, many Americans still thought of themselves, in Jeffersonian terms, as a nation of small farmers—and the men and women who carried out that highly symbolic work were respected as more than just raw material producers. Even as the American economy took a sharp industrial turn at the outset of World War II, *Oklahoma!*—a musical dramatization of farm life—broke Broadway records with its 2,212-show run in the mid-1940s. The film adaptation, released in 1955, won an Academy Award. Stories like *Oklahoma!* struck a chord with many Americans because of the enduring sense that farm people were keepers of our country's agrarian democratic values. Farm families like mine were proud to receive compliments from the people who bought our eggs and cream at the local grocery store.

And yet, for all the attachment to agrarian traditions, the postwar period was also marked by an intense national fascination with progress and modernization. Rural people were not exempt from this fascination—as evidenced by my boyhood speech and debate acquaintances. Even as certain elements of our culture lauded time-honored customs, there were persistent suggestions that our way of life could and should be somehow updated or improved. The popular *Farm Journal* might glorify traditional "country life" with cover images of mothers and daughters canning produce and features on families singing together by candlelight. But peppered throughout the magazine were articles about the advantages of bigger tractors, newer sewing machines, and faster cars. "TV adds so much to farm family happiness," declared one full-page advertisement.[5] This narrative of progress, of course, had been a part of the American agrarian ideal from the very beginnings of the nation. But every generation saw their state of the art as truly new and different, and the postwar push to modernize was promulgated with particular enthusiasm.

I didn't come to see it until much later, but these rival frames of Progress and Tradition did little to help my community of Big Sandy sort out what was and was not valuable among the competing visions of rural economy being debated and experimented with in the postwar years. In many ways, I think *both* of these false utopias made us susceptible to the commodity mindset and cheap food economy, which were just about to deeply transform our community and many like it, bringing us to the brink of collapse. And yet, to this day, pundits concerned about economic decline and political turmoil in places like my hometown frequently offer one or the other of these basic prescriptions—either "go back to the good old days" or modernize. Tragically, we are badly missing the point.

There was nothing magical about the farm machinery or the cropping systems in the Big Sandy of my childhood. In fact, we were doing a lot of things wrong: our tillage was almost certainly too disruptive, we weren't rotating through a diverse enough mix of crops, and we hadn't yet come to understand what we needed to return to the soil to make up for the fertility we were essentially mining. It would be foolish to go back to most of the farming *practices* of that time. But what I think many people in my childhood hometown *did* understand is that there are forms of organizing a community's collective efforts—and the fruits of those efforts—that promote human dignity and provide economic stability. We had not fully realized such an economy, and so long as we relied on selling our harvests into the global commodity system, we never would. But scattered across the landscape in the Big Sandy of my childhood—a microcosm of the postwar transformation of American society—were the seeds of a more honest way to value human lives, the land and communities they depend upon, and the goods that are at once one family's livelihood and another family's quality of life. Those seeds were present at Big Sandy Grain Company *and* the Farmers Union elevator, in the oat-harvesting equipment we shared with our neighbors, both old and new, at the branding parties and the barn raisings. The question for me, then, is not one of tradition or modernity—the question is, Can I sort these promising seeds out? Can I replant and nurture them?

With all the work to be done on the farm during the growing season, summer was not a time for vacations. We did have a few community traditions, however, that we rarely missed: the Memorial Day parade, the Father's Day picnic at the White Rocks along the Missouri River, the Fourth of July picnic and afternoon rodeo in the Bear Paw Mountains—and the county fair in Fort Benton.

My sister and I enjoyed the cotton candy and corn dogs, the Ferris wheel and the Tilt-A-Whirl, the exhibits of crops, animals, and our school art projects from the previous spring. But the real attraction was the chance to see our school friends for the first time in months and catch up on the news and gossip. In the days before cell phones, text messaging, Facebook, and Twitter, the county fair was the center of our social universe.

In late August 1964, I was about to enter my junior year in high school and was attending the county fair as usual. As I approached the exhibit area under the grandstands, I spied an old man with a big red Folger's coffee can filled with grain. "Hey, Sonny," he called over to me, "would you like some of King Tut's wheat?"

I took a couple of steps toward the man, and he grabbed a fistful of kernels out of his coffee can and poured them into my hand. I was amazed by how big they were: three times the size of the wheat we grew on our farm. I thanked the man and put the grain in my pocket, along with a few unused carnival ride tickets and a couple of silver dollars, all of which would soon be gone.

I had no inkling that this grain would, some twenty-five years later, change the whole course of my life.

CHAPTER 2:

Better Farming through Chemistry?

The first time I had a lesson that was called "science" was in the third grade, and I was captivated. As soon as I was old enough, I entered the state science fair, which became one of my favorite events of the year. I still remember my first science fair project: a desalination model made out of glass bowls turned upside down, with a heat lamp over them to mimic the sun. I showed everyone who walked by how the water would condense on the inside of the bowl and run into a trough, transforming seawater into freshwater. I always had an interest in understanding how things work. Especially living things. Science seemed like the key to unlocking the secrets of nature's genius.

After my sophomore year of high school, my parents let me go to a summer science institute at the University of Iowa. They really needed my help on the farm, but they saw that I had a passion for experiments and systematic analysis, so they sent me off to Iowa. I hadn't yet settled on a favorite branch of science, and it hadn't yet occurred to me that my tinkering in the garden was anything scientific. So I chose to focus on math, because I knew that would be important if I wanted to follow in my dad's footsteps as an engineering major. I remember the math being very theoretical, a seemingly endless series of equations on a chalkboard. I had no love for it.

But the next summer, I got to go to a summer science institute again, this time at Virginia Tech, in plant physiology. It was so much fun that I couldn't believe people could get paid to do this kind of thing. This institute focused mostly on applied research: after lectures in the morning, we spent all afternoon working in the lab. We did a number of small experiments on those engrossing afternoons. I remember helping to conduct a rat-feeding study, where we measured the weight gain of rats eating different diets. But my favorite part, by far, was my main research project for the summer, evaluating a new herbicide called dicamba.

My dicamba project involved a combination of outdoor and indoor work. First, I had to go out and dig weeds from the golf course or the roadside. For this experiment, we mainly used plantain—a hardy plant with broad, oval-shaped leaves. After I dug up the plantain plants, I brought them back to the laboratory, where I transferred them into a jar of growing medium for my experiment.

Once the plantain samples were successfully acclimatized to the lab, I put a little solution of dicamba on the leaves. Incorporated into the herbicide was a radioisotope that would allow me to track the chemical's translocation, or movement through the plant. The goal of the research project was to find out where the herbicide went once it was absorbed by the leaves of the plantain. Would it go through the stems into other leaves? Perhaps even down into the roots?

After applying the isotope-tagged dicamba, I waited a few days and then cut the plants into different parts: leaves, stems, roots. Next, I dried out my specimens and put them on x-ray film. My professors at the science institute taught me to develop the x-rays in a darkroom so I could reveal the dark streaks that marked the path of the herbicide. To my amazement, in just a few days, the chemical had translocated throughout the entire plant.

I had no inkling that half a century later dicamba's ability to spread—not just through the plant but also through the air—would devastate midwestern soybean crops, making it the ugly poster child for pesticide drift. I didn't foresee the lawsuits and state government bans, or the violent disputes that would break out between neighbors. I was simply enthralled with the fact that a radioisotope and a sheet of x-ray film could show you what was happening inside a plant, in the mysterious inner sanctums of the xylem and phloem. If this is science, I thought, I want to be a scientist.

By that time, I was going into my senior year of high school, and I came home from my summer science institute hoping to go on to college at Virginia Tech. My dad didn't say much, but I knew he did not really approve of my going out of state. Rather than try to talk me out of it, though, he opted to drive me down to his alma mater, Montana State University in Bozeman, to show me what we had right there in the Big Sky State. After a few discouraging visits to antiquated laboratories that appeared unchanged from the days my father had attended school there, we found a plant pathology lab that had all the same equipment I'd been working with at Virginia Tech. At the helm were two young faculty members, recently graduated from UC Davis, who assured me that they could satisfy my appetite for cutting-edge plant science. I started my bachelor's degree at MSU the next fall, in botany.

My senior year in Bozeman, I took my first class in ecology. The professor was Dr. Collins. I still remember him strolling into class on the first day, cup of coffee in hand, shirt sleeves rolled up. No tie. Unlike many of my other professors—buttoned-down lecturers who had us memorize Latin names and equations—Dr. Collins introduced us to the wonders of nature through a series of gripping stories. He was unlike any authority figure I'd ever met. And he was the first person I knew who called himself an environmentalist.

Of all the stories Dr. Collins told us, the one that had the biggest impact on me was about the eagles in Glacier Park, just a half day's drive from my home in Big Sandy. These magnificent birds were under threat, he explained, because of a poison called DDT. This insecticide had become so prevalent in the environment, he explained, that low levels were being taken up by plankton, the tiny organisms at the bottom of the food chain in Northwest Montana's Flathead Lake. When these plankton were eaten by salmon, the poison accumulated, and when the salmon were eaten by eagles, the poison concentrated even further, to the point where it interfered with the eagles' calcium metabolism. As a result, the birds were laying eggs with paper-thin shells—or no shells at all.[1]

I had been in high school when Rachel Carson's *Silent Spring* came out, and I had a basic awareness that DDT was toxic. I had sprayed it in our bunkhouse one time to kill the flies, and I still remember the nasty headache I had afterward. But insecticides like DDT weren't widely used in Montana grain agriculture, which had the advantage of cold winters to take care of most insect pests. So my early exposure to Rachel Carson's book never really caused me to question farming practices or the herbicides and fertilizers my dad used. My image of environmentalism was still a bunch of hippies in California protesting industrial pollution.

Until I met this ecology professor. He was the first one in my life to get me thinking about the seriousness of environmental degradation in ways that called into question what *farmers* were doing. I listened carefully, but even then, I didn't connect the dots back to my own family's wheat farm. I still thought about it in terms of big farms in California or the Midwest that were using a lot of insecticides, and maybe a few produce farmers up near Glacier Park who were spraying the same stuff. It wasn't *our* problem.

After I finished my bachelor's and master's degrees in botany at Bozeman, my professors encouraged me to go on for a PhD at the same university where they had studied: UC Davis. The hot new field in plant science at the time was plant biochemistry, and Davis had one of the leading programs. The university, one of the premier ag schools in the world, was also a key driver of the "green revolution"—an ambitious campaign to raise crop yields through new scientific breeding techniques and the use of chemical fertilizers and pesticides. I applied and was accepted. I moved to Davis in 1971 with my new bride, Ann, a local Bozeman girl with whom one of my professors had set me up on a blind date.

I liked a lot of things about UC Davis. I was still fascinated with the inner workings of plants, and my degree program gave me eye-opening new insights into the botanical world: proteins, carbohydrates, lipids. When we charted the series of chemical reactions occurring within the cells of a plant, these metabolic pathways stretched out across the chalkboard like maps of an increasingly familiar landscape, the names of towns and roads along the way becoming second nature. As I furthered my studies, I came to a deep appreciation for the magnificent order of the universe and the interrelations that characterized living systems. I found it quite inspiring to see how everything was tied to everything else.

My most memorable learning experiences, however, happened outside the classroom: on field trips. In the fertile valleys south of San Francisco, I saw fields upon fields of artichokes, a crop we couldn't grow in Montana. In the arid country east of San Diego, I saw the massive irrigation pipes that coaxed lettuce, oranges, and date palms from these desert soils. Having been raised in a place with a four-month growing season, I found the diversity of California agriculture nothing short of marvelous. And, of course, the camaraderie of sharing these excursions with my fellow students from all over the world was wonderful. But the lab work wasn't as much fun as I'd expected.

The UC Davis biochemistry department was ranked among the top ten in the country and wanted to be in the top five. It was that kind of mentality—very competitive. I was stunned when we visited colleagues at a nearby school and were told not to share information about our research, since they were competing with us for the same grant money. The greater goal of advancing science for the public good kind of fell by the wayside, or so it seemed to me.

Despite my discouragement with the politics of the academic research establishment, I completed my PhD in 1976. I considered a career path focused on teaching, and I was also encouraged to explore lucrative opportunities available in the agricultural industry. One of my classmates went to work for a large chemical company that was expanding its work in biotechnology, which was rapidly escalating the green revolution into a gene revolution. It was called Monsanto.

At the time, I didn't question biotechnology. There was a lab across the hall from mine that was doing some early experiments with these genetically modified organisms, or GMOs. They were trying to take a protein from arctic fish and put it into plants to reduce their susceptibility to frost. That seemed to me like a very interesting and noble idea and a natural extension of plant science.

I didn't imagine any kind of corporate control mechanism that would go along with that, like we've seen with the introduction of GMO crops—where farmers can no longer replant their own seed and these companies can patent life. I didn't foresee the centralization of seeds and power and money that's come of having over 90 percent of corn and soybeans and canola dominated by these GMO varieties.[2] I didn't think about GMO traits cross-pollinating and contaminating other plants. Or a GMO that would one day cause a firestorm of controversy surrounding dicamba, the herbicide I had studied at the Virginia Tech summer science institute.[3]

None of those concerns were part of the discussion. The discussion was, How can we make these plants more cold tolerant, like this fish in the Arctic? He's got a protein that keeps him from freezing. Let's see if we can transfer that into a plant. Wouldn't that be a great way to save plants from perishing in an unexpected frost?

But I did have another experience while I was at Davis that started me questioning the so-called modern trajectory of American agriculture. This was the fateful trip to the Central Valley peach farm that transformed the entire course of my career.

When my professor and the peach farmer started laughing about the way these peaches were "ripened"—using a petroleum-based spray developed by the professor that changed their color artificially—I was horrified. For as long as humans had been eating peaches, people had relied on their senses to tell when the fruit was ripe and to judge its quality. That's how we'd sized up peaches when I was a kid: if it looked good, it was. Now two unscrupulous profiteers were poised to change all that, denying the rest of us not only quality, ripe peaches but even the ability to know one when we saw one. My disgust only deepened as I realized the punch line of their joke was how they'd buried the results of their trials in an obscure journal overseas to avoid public scrutiny. This wasn't the science I'd fallen in love with as a youth, the science that endeavored to uncover the inner workings of nature's genius for the benefit of humanity. This was manipulative. Literally tasteless. And potentially harmful.

On that field trip to the Central Valley, I saw that the agriculture I was being trained in, industrial agriculture, was undermining fundamental human values. Honesty, for one. But also respect for the natural world and for the interconnections among living systems that I was just beginning to grasp. Nutrition, taste, and environmental stewardship were all being sacrificed to an economic logic that I couldn't understand and didn't particularly want to. But one thing was patently clear: this new direction was not about meeting human needs; it was about increasing markets and profits—in total disregard of the quality of the end product.

Somewhere between my horror over those rock-hard peaches and my frustration with the cutthroat competition over grants, any remaining ambition I might have had to become a research scientist sort of fizzled. I didn't apply for any postdoctoral fellowships, and I never looked for one of those high-paying jobs in Big Ag. Instead, I ended up starting a small business with a friend, supplying biological products to hospital laboratories and conducting contract research. A few years in, we merged with a more established contract research business that specialized in drug and alcohol analysis, and we started earning regular salaries.

After the merger, we did less work with hospitals and a lot more forensic studies related to legal proceedings. Alcohol levels in blood samples, identification of drugs seized by law enforcement, that sort of stuff. We would conduct our analysis, bring our results to court, sit in the hallway while the lawyers made backroom deals, and wait until they gave us the high sign that everything was settled and told us to go home. It was less than satisfying.

When we did make it into the courtroom, it wasn't much better. Nobody actually wanted to know what we'd found. The defense lawyers just wanted to make us look like fools. Their first objective was to protect their client by discrediting our analysis, so they tried to convince the jury that I didn't know what I was doing.

"How long have you been in your current position?" they'd start in, innocently enough. "Do you have specific training to do this type of lab analysis?" But on the next question they went for the jugular. "What is your highest level of education?" they would ask, striking a condescending posture to remind the jury that they were an expert with a JD, while I was likely a lab tech who might have been to community college. As a scientist, I didn't mind close scrutiny of my analytic process. But when I saw that the lawyers were trying to cast doubt on my work by denigrating me as a person, it made me question the fairness of our judicial system.

After one too many experiences like that, I got frustrated and smarted off to one of those lawyers. He was asking me how many hours I'd spent in the lab and whether I'd ever seen this kind of chemical analysis equipment before I started working for the contract research company. His tone was maddeningly disdainful, as though he were talking to a kindergartner. I told the lawyer I had a PhD from UC Davis, and then I added a smart-alecky question: "Do you think that's enough?" I doubt I said it in a very polite tone of voice. The judge told my boss that if I said anything like that again he would hold me in contempt. I was told to be respectful, answer the question, and not make any editorial comments.

The courtroom atmosphere started to wear me down. The lawyers were totally impenetrable to me—they had no sense of humor, and they didn't seem to have any interest in justice. Their job was to find loopholes to get their clients set free. Meanwhile, my role in the judicial process didn't feel like a meaningful contribution either. Why even conduct these forensic analyses when most cases were settled without even consulting them?

In the midst of this turmoil, I found myself deep in prayer one day, asking what I should do next. Academia didn't seem to be for me. But my business wasn't very fulfilling either. I had just turned thirty, and my wife and I had three young daughters, who would soon be starting school. I needed some answers.

All of a sudden, in a moment that truly felt like divine guidance, a solution came to me in the form of a still, small voice. Now was the time for me to return home.

My wife was surprised when I broached the idea, but she liked the thought of being closer to her parents, who still lived in Montana. Farming was a new thing for her—she was a city girl from college-town Bozeman—but she told me she'd be willing to give it a try. Then I called my dad, and he more or less offered to hand over the tractor keys on the spot. Within a few months, my folks showed up with a grain truck full of wheat. We sold the wheat in California, packed up the grain truck with all our stuff, squeezed ourselves and our three daughters into our old Chevy, and headed north.

CHAPTER 3:

Beyond Commodities

When I returned to Big Sandy in 1978, I found a very different town from the one where I had grown up. The pool hall and the soda foun tain where we used to order root beer floats after school were gone. The theater where my friends and I had watched *To Kill a Mockingbird* and shared ten-cent bags of popcorn had burned down, and it was never replaced.

As I drove out to my family's farm, I noticed that many of the houses along the road were empty, with weeds growing up around them. The fields were bigger, and so was the farm machinery parked alongside them. I was accustomed to seeing farmers plant their hilliest ground in alternating strips of grain and fallow, as we'd all been encouraged to do by the Soil Conservation Service, to prevent erosion. But as I surveyed the massive fields that now surrounded Big Sandy, I saw that nearly all these strips had been taken out. Our farm was no different.

Between 1950 and 1997, the American countryside lost more than 3 million family farms, and with them went much of rural society.[1] With the exodus of farmers came the failure of many small businesses, which no longer had the support they needed to keep their doors open.

Communities that had once been vibrant places to live came to resemble outdoor factories, with large tracts of land managed by a handful of overworked farmers who no longer had many places—or much time—to gather and socialize. The decline of my community—and thousands of other rural communities across the United States—was not an accident. Moving people off farms and consolidating farmland to more efficiently produce cheap commodities was explicit government policy.

In 1962, when I was still in high school, an influential group of American businessmen released a report titled "An Adaptive Program for Agriculture." Unbeknownst to me and likely most other folks at the time, this report spelled out the rural policy favored by this economic think tank, which was headed by powerful executives from Ford Motor Company and Sears. They had chosen an innocuous name for themselves: the Committee for Economic Development. But their vision of the American economy was one in which manufacturing interests, concentrated in the hands of powerful men like themselves, dominated. The primary role of production agriculture in such an economy would be to produce inexpensive raw materials for urban food processors. These processors would produce cheap food for the laboring masses needed to work in urban factories—whose ranks would be recruited from the "surplus" rural population: "excess" farmers no longer needed to manage increasingly streamlined operations and "unnecessary" small businesses that served these farm communities. "Agriculture's chief need is a reduction of the number of people," the Committee for Economic Development declared in its 1962 report. They recommended "getting a large number of people out of agriculture before they are committed to it as a career."[2]

By the time I was a graduate student at UC Davis, in the early 1970s, the committee's vision had become the official party line at the US Department of Agriculture, where Secretary Earl Butz urged farmers to "get big or get out" because "agriculture is big business." Butz was heavily involved in crafting farm programs and subsidies that gave larger farms an advantage over smaller ones.[3] When farmers protested the destructive impacts that such "economic development" was having on their communities—reduced farm incomes, increased farm debt, loss of community infrastructure as towns emptied out—Butz told them to "adapt or die."[4]

The Committee for Economic Development was successful in getting a large number of people out of agriculture and consolidating farms, throughout both Democratic and Republican administrations. The American farm population declined by 26 percent between 1960 and 1970[5] and continued to fall as Butz took the helm of the USDA in 1971. In order to farm more acres and produce more food with less labor, farmers purchased larger machinery and relied heavily on chemical fertilizers and pesticides. This was good for the manufacturing industry that the Committee for Economic Development sought to boost: by the 1970s, more than 100 industrial plants were producing approximately 1,000 agricultural chemicals, which would then be combined into more than 50,000 registered pesticides.[6]

For farmers, however, high-input, high-volume commodity agriculture meant steadily increasing debt. In the seventeen-year period before I returned to the farm, American farm debt had jumped by 400 percent.[7] Some of my parents' neighbors were forced to sell farms that had been in their families for three generations. And our own annual "operating note"—the money we borrowed from the bank to run the farm—grew larger and larger, becoming harder and harder to repay at the end of each season.

Individual farm debt wasn't the only indicator that commodity agriculture was a losing proposition for much of rural America. The loss of individual economic security was bad enough, but the most troubling trend I witnessed upon my return to Big Sandy was the loss of infrastructure, institutions, and relationships: the fundamental things that held our community together. The country dances had disappeared, as had the community picnics along the river. There were fewer businesses on Main Street.

A USDA anthropologist named Walter Goldschmidt had seen this coming and had gone to California in the 1940s to study how the industrialization of farms impacted rural communities. As I'd witnessed firsthand at Davis, California agriculture had industrialized decades before the USDA began calling for grain farmers in America's heartland to follow suit, and it was thus a potential canary in the coal mine. Goldschmidt's findings were devastating. Comparing an industrialized agricultural area with one that had not yet followed the "get big or get out" mantra, he found a smaller middle class, lower incomes, higher poverty rates, poorer-quality schools, and fewer community institutions: civic organizations, churches, and retail businesses. Furthermore, residents of the industrialized agricultural area had less control over public decisions as outside agribusiness interests flexed their political muscle.[8]

Future research would corroborate Goldschmidt's findings and add other deleterious social impacts of industrial agriculture: unemployment, crime, depression, diminished civic participation, even a reduction in the degree to which rural people trusted one another.[9] I saw this in my own hometown: as the bigger farms bought out the smaller farms, our neighbors disappeared until half the families whose kids I'd gone to school with were gone. Ostensibly, we remaining farmers were supposed to benefit from our increased production, but it was pretty clear that value was predominantly traveling one way: *out*. Still, higher-ups at Goldschmidt's agency pressed on with their strategy for economic development: cheap commodities. Earl Butz wasn't the first to push such policies, nor would he be the last.

As the USDA pushed headlong into its "adaptive program" for agriculture, American farms lost more than just people. In the rush to maximize production of commodities—in our area, wheat and barley—a host of other plants and animals that supplied critical nutrients to farms and their surrounding communities vanished. In 1950, over 78 percent of American farms had poultry. More than 67 percent had dairy cattle. Nearly 56 percent had hogs. By 1997, these numbers would dwindle to 5 percent, 6.1 percent, and 5.7 percent, respectively. Produce followed a similar trajectory: in 1950, nearly 29 percent of American farms produced apples; by 1997, that figure was down to 1.5 percent.[10] The diversification my dad had always practiced—so that we could have a more stable income, cycle some of our own nutrients, adapt to unpredictable weather and markets, and provide our own fresh milk, meat, and eggs—was becoming a thing of the past. In the process, farms like ours were sacrificing much of their ecological, nutritional, and economic value, becoming more and more dependent on chemical inputs and commodity markets.

By the time I returned to my parents' farm in 1978, the social and economic pain of rural America had reached a pressure point. Six months before I came home, on December 10, 1977, farmers drove their tractors to a number of state capitols, demanding an end to legislation benefiting agribusiness at the expense of family farms. A year later, a large tractorcade stopped traffic in Washington, DC.[11] I began to realize that the difficulties I'd heard about from my parents weren't unique to our community, nor were they the usual cyclical downturns of markets or weather. The very viability of family farming in the United States was at stake.

By the late 1970s and early 1980s, life on the farm was very different from what it had been in my childhood. Gone were the days of sharing equipment. Our neighbors took out big loans and bought larger machinery to handle their ever-increasing acreages. A new combine (short for "combination harvester-thresher," the machine that most American grain farmers use to harvest their crop) was now a $100,000 investment. Farm women, who in my mother's day had been active participants in the productive activities of the household—putting up food for the winter, overseeing the family garden, and helping with the grain harvest—disappeared from the fields and the homesteads. With farm incomes falling short of meeting rural families' needs, these women commuted to work in towns as far as an hour's drive away, leaving their husbands with even more to do. Everyone seemed to be behind, racing to keep up with the bills and the chores. Conversations were becoming a rare luxury.

In California's Central Valley, I'd seen that industrial agriculture was becoming further and further removed from any sort of concern with the people who ate the food. Back home in Montana, I saw that this "modern" agriculture was even less concerned with the people who grew it. Consequently, the profession of farming had lost a bit of its luster as the noble cornerstone of Jeffersonian American democracy, and it was becoming rare for young people like me to return home. People didn't brag about their son who came home and drove a tractor. They bragged about their son who went off to medical school or got a high-paying job at the bank.

I wasn't terribly concerned with the prestige factor, but I had an undeniable financial problem. My parents' 2,400 acres—an average-size Montana family farm in those days—was too small to support two families in the era of industrial commodity agriculture. My dad was still eight years away from getting Social Security payments, and I now had four children, with a fifth yet to come. We needed more income.

The thought of trying to keep up by buying out the neighbors didn't appeal to me at all. I didn't want to go into that much debt, and I didn't want to lose my neighbors. So instead of trying to expand, I tried to think of an enterprise that could add value to the farm we already had.

Given my background in plant biochemistry and my few years of experience running lab analyses for courts in California, my first thought was to set up a lab and offer a soil-testing service. I had business cards printed up for the Triangle Research Center, and I ordered a soil-testing kit. But then it became painfully obvious that the time of year I needed to run all those soil tests was the same time of year I needed to be seeding my own crops, in both fall and spring.

While I was trying to figure out my next move, my fourth cousin came up from Southern California for a visit. He was out of a job and thought he might start a business selling pheasants to high-end restaurants in California. He asked me what I thought. I'd known of only one pheasant farm, I told him. A group of people in our neighborhood had tried it a few years prior, and their business had ended when foxes got in and ate all the birds.

I told my cousin I had a different idea. How about finding me some California customers for my wheat? This was my first notion about how I could add some value back to my family's farm production: by side-stepping the large-scale grain-handling and -milling industry and selling premium-quality whole grain directly to bakers.

I knew there was a good market in California for premium whole grain because I had sold a little bit of my family's wheat to a nearby bakery when I was still living there.

I'd had a friend who was in law school at UC Davis in the early 1970s. He was the first person who told me about organic food. He went on and on about how organic agriculture was growing healthier plants and was a better way to farm. I thought, What is this guy in law school doing, trying to tell me about agriculture? I'm a plant biochemist, raised on a farm. I didn't believe him. I didn't accept it. I just responded the way I always do when I don't really want to say what I am thinking: "That's very interesting."

It was a good thing I kept the conversation going, though, because my law student friend went on to tell me that there was a mill in South

San Francisco that bought grain directly from farmers. They were making premium whole grain bread, and they were looking for high-protein wheat.

The miller's name turned out to be Al Giusto, and he was a genial guy. Even over the phone, I could tell that he was the kind of person who took his work seriously but didn't take himself too seriously. Businesslike but friendly, he was passionate about high-quality bread.

Al knew that Montana was a good place to source high-protein wheat, but he didn't have any connections in the Big Sky State. So the next time my parents visited me in California, we all went down to Al's mill and bakery. My folks were polite but no-nonsense—both had been in the navy before returning to the Montana farm where my father had grown up, and they both wore the same plain, boxy-framed glasses. My father, Mack, wore his cowboy hat and a nice flannel shirt, and he liked to hear hard numbers before anybody tried to win him over with pleasantries. But Al immediately impressed my mother, Dordy, with homemade coconut macaroons—which became a tradition on all our subsequent visits to his plant.

Right there in that first meeting, Al offered to pay a dollar per bushel above conventional prices for my family's high-protein wheat. He even offered to pay for the grain to get cleaned and bagged. There was a facility near Big Sandy to do the cleaning and the bagging, so that was not a long haul for us, and this new market probably increased the value of my dad's crop by 20 or 30 percent. It was a huge boon.

Honestly, at that time, that's really all it was: we were growing a premium product, and we found a market that would pay us a premium price. I didn't eat whole wheat. I didn't think about health. One time, Al asked us about organic. I told him our wheat was nearly as good as organic because we used herbicide only once per season, and some years not at all. Other than that, I told Al, the only chemical we used was fertilizer, and there were no signs of it in the plant or the grain.

What I told Al was what I'd been taught at Davis, and at Bozeman before that: a plant can't tell the difference between nitrogen from a fertilizer sack and nitrogen from a barnyard manure pile. That's what I believed.

I could tell by Al's facial expressions and body language that he wasn't buying my line. But he was still interested in buying my dad's wheat, for his non-organic bread, so I let it go.

For two years my dad sold wheat to Al Giusto, and when I came back home to the farm, I was hoping to keep that relationship going. But the year after I got back to Big Sandy, I sent Al our samples and he didn't buy anything. Four winters came and went without any phone calls from California. I wasn't living there anymore, and with four kids and a farm to run, I wasn't in a position to go back just to try to hunt up new business. But my cousin was.

Once I'd talked him out of the pheasant venture, I suggested that he do some sleuthing around when he returned home to Southern California and see if he couldn't find some customers down there like Al: whole grain bakeries that were looking for high-protein wheat.

My cousin headed off on his quest, and within a few days he called and told me he'd found a guy who wanted a truckload of wheat per week. I found a facility in Fort Benton that was willing to clean our grain. Then I found a trucker in Great Falls whose main route was hauling vegetables north from California to big cities in Western Canada, and he offered us a bargain price to deliver our product on his way back south, as his backhaul. We were in business. In the fall of 1983, my cousin and I officially founded two sister companies, both called the Montana Wheat Company. Mine, based in Montana, was charged with production and procurement of high-quality whole grain wheat. My cousin's company, based in California, would focus on customer service and marketing.

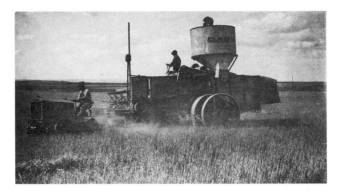

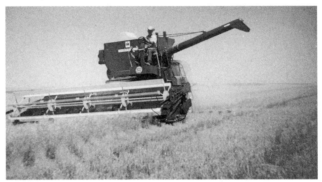

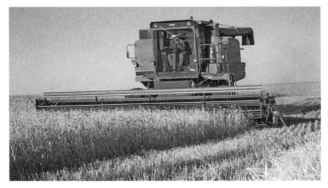

THREE GENERATIONS OF HARVEST. AT THE TOP, MY GRANDFATHER PULLS HIS
COMBINE BEHIND A TRACTOR. IN THE MIDDLE, MY DAD OPERATES HIS NEW
SELF-PROPELLING INTERNATIONAL HARVESTER COMBINE, CIRCA 1960.
AT THE BOTTOM, I HARVEST MY KAMUT CROP FROM THE COMFORT OF AN
AIR-CONDITIONED CAB.
(Top two photos courtesy of Bob Quinn, bottom photo by Hilary Page)

We got started with that one load of wheat per week. Then we picked up another one and another one, until the demand outstripped the supply from my farm and I started sourcing from some of my neighbors too. When I looked at the numbers at the end of the first year, I realized I had almost doubled my income. It was quite low at the time, so it wasn't hard to double, but it was just what we were looking for. Growing high-quality wheat and selling it directly to buyers, whole, was an enterprise that could help support two families on one farm.

There are three main components in a grain of wheat. The majority of the fiber resides in the nutrient-rich outer coating known as the bran. Essential fatty acids abound in the germ, the living embryo that would sprout into a new wheat plant were you to sow the seed. Together, bran and germ contain most of the grain's iron, vitamins, and antioxidants. But the majority of the calories are in the largest, starchiest component: the endosperm.[12]

People have had a taste for endosperm since ancient times. As far back as the Roman Empire, bakers painstakingly attempted to sift the prized starch out from the other components of wheat flour, producing expensive "white" bread—a fashionable luxury food for the wealthy.[13] This sifting process was not without its critics: the ancient Greek philosopher Plato registered concerns about the nutritional value of refined flour in his *Republic*.[14] But the ancients' white bread was nothing like the cellophane-wrapped supermarket loaves we see today. Sifting eliminated only the largest chunks of bran, so much of this fibrous coating and nearly all of the oily germ remained.[15]

Until, that is, the nineteenth-century arrival of the steel roller mill, which finally shaved the endosperm cleanly away from both bran and germ.[16] Just one small hurdle stood in the way of truly white flour: the beta-carotene (the precursor to vitamin A) that tinted refined wheat slightly yellow. Industrial processors discovered that exposing the flour to gusts of chlorine gas could eliminate that.[17] Flour—and the panoply of products that would soon be made from it—was now pure, gleaming white starch. It could be stored for years.[18]

Picking up where Plato left off, a group of French and British doctors and medical experts raised concerns about the nutritional value of this white flour, noting the nutrient deficiencies and chronic diseases that appeared to follow in its wake.[19] Joining this chorus of warnings against white bread was Sylvester Graham, a Presbyterian minister and health food crusader whose 1837 *Treatise on Bread and Bread-Making* converted many leading public intellectuals of the day to whole grain diets, including Henry David Thoreau.[20] Thoreau followed Graham's dietary advice religiously while at Walden Pond and saw it as central to his project of social reform. The transcendentalist author even paraphrased Graham's work on bread in the text of his classic book *Walden*, recommending that his readers grow their own wheat and grind it in a handmill.[21] In the early twentieth century, Graham's ideas were revived by brothers Will and John Kellogg, who manufactured the first graham cracker and went on to develop America's first mass-market line of breakfast cereals based on Graham's ideas.[22] The biggest push for whole grain, however, came in the 1940s, when 30 percent of the men originally drafted for service in World War II were turned away for diet-related physical deficiencies. A national campaign to improve nutrition ensued, and it appeared white bread might be doomed.[23] The refined loaves, wrote leading pure food campaigner Dr. Harvey Wiley, were "white and waxy as the face of a corpse."[24]

But legislating whole grain would have undermined the business model of the burgeoning food-processing industry, which relied on standardized, shelf-stable ingredients. So instead, politicians were persuaded to adopt the solution proffered by another charismatic doctor by the name of Russell Wilder: injecting white bread with added vitamins such as thiamine. Rather than going out of business, industrial bakers now had a new market opportunity as they were called upon to "solve" the problem they had created. By the middle of World War II, 75 percent of the country's bread was thus "enriched," and public relations experts were already perfecting the art of persuading Americans that value was being added to their bread rather than subtracted from it.[25]

Whole grain bread and flour were relegated to the shelves of idiosyncratic health food stores until the late 1960s, when a generation of counterculture activists began raising concerns about the corporate food system. These activists were concerned about the nutrient content of their own diets—and deeply distrustful of the preservatives and other additives used in industrial food processing. Many were influenced by macrobiotics, a natural food philosophy based on Zen Buddhism, which taught that whole grains should be at the center of the diet.[26] But the counterculture was even more concerned about lining the pockets of the increasingly concentrated processed food sector, which they saw as part of a military-industrial complex undermining the democratic foundation of American society.[27] In the attempt to create an alternative "people's food system," they formed cooperative grocery stores, purchased whole grains in bulk,[28] and spurred a large-scale revival in home baking that spread well beyond college towns and hippie enclaves into the American mainstream.[29] They also formed cooperative bakeries with names like Uprisings and Rebel Bakers Collective.[30]

By the late 1970s, a growing number of these cooperative bakeries and grocery stores not only wanted to buy whole grain; they wanted to buy it directly from family farmers. But beyond a handful of pioneering companies like Little Bear Trading Company in Minnesota and Arrowhead Mills in Texas, they struggled to find sources. So my cousin and I decided to focus our business on serving these renegades: bakers who wanted to work with real, complex, whole grain.

Given that we were seeking out independent-minded whole grain bakers in California, it wasn't long before I heard the "O" word again. In fact, our original customer soon asked us if we could supply him with organically grown wheat. It was 1984. I didn't know a single organic farmer in Montana.

When Al Giusto had first asked me about organic in 1976, I could afford to be dismissive because my little grain deal with him was just a side business I was doing to help out my dad. But by 1984, selling grain to bakeries was quite literally my bread and butter, and I'd happened to carve out a niche in a Southern California crowd that might just find another supplier if I couldn't come up with organic. So I hunted all over Montana to see what I could find.

I finally found a farmer in the northeast corner of the state who was growing wheat organically and was willing to sell me some so I could supply it to my customer in California. But in those days, Montana didn't have a law defining what "organic" was. So I had the farmer sign an affidavit saying he was in compliance with all the stipulations of the organic labeling law California had at that time: no pesticides or fertilizers for two years before harvest of the organic crop, and no chemical treatment on the seed. From that first sale, the organic side of my business grew steadily: within four years, nearly half the grain I was shipping down to California would be organic.

I didn't think the affidavit system was a great way to do business, though, and our customers didn't either. So I got on board with an effort to write an organic definition statute for Montana, which became the fourth state in the nation to pass such a law, in 1985. In the process, I became acquainted with the pioneers of organic agriculture in our area, people like David Oien in Conrad, Montana, Fred Kirschenmann in North Dakota, and Fred's mentor, David Vetter, from Nebraska.

I was amazed by the enthusiasm these organic farmers had for what they were doing. I had never seen anything like that at the Montana

Grain Growers meetings or the Farm Bureau gatherings. Those farmers were all worried about commodity prices going down or trying to figure out how to get more out of the government programs. I was hearing very little upbeat talk among conventional farmers in the late 1980s, a period historians now call the "farm crisis." The cost of chemical inputs was soaring just as grain prices stagnated, all in the midst of a drought and a precipitous drop in land values across the Midwest. It was survival mode.

But the organic farmers were a totally different breed. They were excited and hopeful about the future. Go-getters. Doers. Problem solvers. Scientists, really. These were my kind of folks.

I loved the idea of a farming system that didn't require herbicides. After my childhood experiences watching my garden plants curl up and die from the 2,4-D wafting off my dad's clothing when he walked by after spraying, I'd been haunted by the thought of what those chemicals might be doing to human health. When I came back to the farm, my mom and dad moved to town and I took over all the chores. Except one. Spraying. I let my dad do that because I figured he was done having kids.

But fertilizers were a different story. When I came back to the farm I still believed what I'd been taught at Davis and had tried to explain to Al Giusto. Nitrogen is one of the three key macronutrients necessary for plant growth. It is abundant in the atmosphere, but it has to be converted into a different form in order for plants to take it up and use it. For most of human history, farmers had two options for securing this "plant-available" nitrogen. They could apply animal manure or compost to their fields, or they could rotate their grain crops with legumes, a family of plants capable of "fixing" nitrogen. These legumes—lentils, chickpeas, alfalfa, and their cousins—teamed up with soil bacteria to convert atmospheric nitrogen into a form they could use as fertilizer. Then they left some behind for the grains that followed them in the field.

In the early twentieth century, two clever guys named Fritz Haber and Carl Bosch figured out a chemical process that allowed them to transform nitrogen into a plant-available form in a factory so farmers would no longer have to rely on manure and nitrogen-fixing plants. This nitrogen-synthesizing process won the 1918 Nobel Prize for Chemistry. At the molecular level, synthetic nitrogen created by the Haber-Bosch process and delivered in a fertilizer bag is no different from organic nitrogen delivered by manure and beans. The plants don't care how they get their nitrogen. So why should we?

My new friends in the organic farming community explained the holes in this logic. I was thinking of plants strictly in terms of my graduate training in chemistry, but I needed to draw a little more on my undergraduate training in biology. Yes, plants need nitrogen. But to be healthy and weather tough times, they need more than just nitrogen—they also need organic matter, the living fraction of the soil. Microscopic soil life supports plants in numerous ways, from stimulating their growth to detoxifying harmful chemicals to suppressing disease.[31] The situation under the ground, I realized, was much like the one above it. When the USDA told farmers to get big or get out, my family had balked, knowing that in the long haul, we needed the ongoing support of our neighbors more than a fleeting influx of capital. The same principle held true for our plants—a onetime boost of synthetic nitrogen fertilizer was no substitute for the ongoing support provided by a community of symbiotic organisms.

When farmers fertilize with manure and legumes, they continually add organic matter back to the farm at the same time, stimulating billions of microbes living in the soil. Not so with Haber-Bosch nitrogen. In fact, long-term use of chemical fertilizer actually depletes soil organic matter—and decreases microbial activity.[32] After a few decades, you're essentially farming dead soil.

By the mid-1980s, the consequences of starving out soil life were becoming evident across much of the grain belt. More inputs were needed to boost yields and grain quality. And to add insult to injury, dead soil doesn't hold water very well, so when drought hit hard in the latter half of the decade—sending most of the Midwest and Great Plains into the worst downturn in farming since the Great Depression—the plants didn't have a moisture reserve to draw on. Farmers poured more and more nitrogen fertilizer on, but with ever-diminishing financial returns. Herbicides were a similar story: the more we used, the more our weeds developed resistance. We were on a chemical treadmill.

Fortunately for me, there was a way to get off that treadmill, and it started with an attitude adjustment. I used to think the farmer's job was to feed the plant. But my new friends in the organic community taught me that the real job of the farmer is to feed the soil. Then the soil feeds the plant. If you focus on feeding the plant, you're thinking only about this year. If you focus on feeding the soil, you're investing in the health of your farm for years to come. The first approach is extractive and short-term. The second approach is regenerative and long-term.

When I started selling my wheat directly to whole grain bakeries, for a price based on quality, I took the first step toward adding value back to my wheat. But it was just a first step. Now that I'd figured out how to bypass industrial processing, I needed to follow the supply chain back two stages further. The final step would come once I realized how drastically the commodity food system had altered our seeds. But in the meantime, I needed to take a hard look at what I was doing in my own fields. I needed to see for myself if organic agriculture could really work on the dry prairie of north central Montana.

CHAPTER 4:

Going Organic

In the fall of 1986, I launched my first experiment with organic. I prepared two twenty-acre fields for winter wheat planting, side by side. The first field would be chemical free. I had been growing alfalfa hay there for the past few years, so I hadn't been spraying it with herbicide. And since alfalfa is a legume, I had plowed it into the soil in place of synthetic fertilizer. I took a soil test to measure how much nitrogen I got from the alfalfa and found that it was pretty high: ninety-five pounds per acre.

The second field was my control. To be sure it was an apples-to-apples comparison, we took soil tests to see how much nitrogen was present. Since we hadn't planted legumes there for some time, we weren't surprised to find that the nitrogen content was significantly lower than in the field that had been planted with alfalfa. But we didn't want to give the organic experiment an unfair advantage, so we added enough synthetic nitrogen fertilizer to the control plot to make sure both fields had an equivalent start at ninety-five pounds per acre.

The only difference between the two fields was the row spacing of the seeds. In the control field, I planted the rows of wheat seeds fourteen inches apart, as we normally did. But in the organic field, I planted them closer together, just seven inches apart. I had been told that getting quick canopy cover—smothering out any unwanted plants with a consistent stand of crops that captured all the sunlight—was important for preventing weed problems in organic systems. So, in essence, I used the narrower row spacing to substitute for the herbicide that we used in the control field.

As the ground began to freeze in the late fall, the wheat seedlings in both fields "hardened off," pausing their growth to wait out the cold Montana winter. I could hardly wait for the snow to melt so I could see how the two fields would develop the following spring.

We had some unusual late summer rain the next year, which stimulated the growth of something we didn't want: kochia, otherwise known as fireweed. To make matters worse, the weed outbreak came after we'd already sprayed all our conventional fields with herbicide, as we typically did in late May. Since we were able to spray only one time, there was nothing we could do but watch the fireweed grow and worry about it. By the time August rolled around, there were so many kochia plants in the control field that they interfered with the harvest, and we had to be careful that they didn't plug up the combine or put too much moisture into the wheat and cause it to mold in storage. Slowly, carefully, I harvested the two fields and gathered my data.

The yields from the organic and conventional fields were nearly identical. So was the protein content. And the chemical field was weedier than the organic one! The narrow row spacing in our experimental plot had shaded out the kochia plants, and they never got started. My father was astounded. He'd spent hundreds of thousands of dollars on fertilizer and herbicide—only to find out that he could have accomplished the same thing by strategically growing alfalfa at the right time in his crop rotation and planting his wheat seeds closer together.

Starting with those twenty acres in 1986, I transitioned our farm to organic very rapidly. The spring of 1988, just my second growing season "experimenting" with organic, turned out to be the last time I ever used chemicals on a single acre of the farm.

The summer of 1988 brought a disastrous drought. Our wheat plants were short and shriveled, and many failed to develop so much as a single kernel of grain. We didn't even bother to harvest some of our conventional fields—the yield on my twenty-acre control plot from the previous season, for example, was zero. My organic field was nothing to brag about—four bushels per acre. But it was enough to pay for the cost of harvesting, with a little profit on top. From the perspective of gross yields, you might say it was a small but significant difference.

But if you looked at 1988 from the perspective of net profit, the difference between the organic field and the chemical field was night and day. My only expense for the organic field was the seed, and I got enough crop to get my seed back. But I'd put a lot of money into the fertilizer and sprays for the chemical field and I still got zero. It was a huge loss. The thing was, I didn't actually have to pay my chemical bill. The federal government was essentially covering it for me.

When I started my transition to organic, I began paying more attention to our crop subsidies, because they were getting smaller. In those days, subsidy payments were calculated on "base acres"—the number of acres a farmer had enrolled and committed to use for a particular crop. You couldn't get base acres for just any crop, only the ones the federal government had included in its commodity program. Midwesterners mostly had them for corn and soybeans, which they had sufficient rain and sunshine to grow. In the South, people had base acres in cotton. But in our area, the only options were wheat and barley. Organic farming required more diverse cropping rotations than just wheat and barley to properly feed the soil and break up pest cycles, so I was gradually taking our farm out of base acres to grow a wider variety of crops, thus forgoing some of our subsidies.

Curious to see what I was missing out on, I looked up the size of our subsidy payments from the mid-1980s, right before I started transitioning to organic. They ranged from about $24,000 to $26,000 per year. Then I looked up our annual chemical bills. They also ranged from about $24,000 to $26,000 per year. The government subsidy was paying our chemical bill! No wonder nobody bothered to think about how to reduce it. The whole sorry system was propped up at the taxpayer's expense. Worst of all, American taxpayers weren't even subsidizing family farmers, as they no doubt believed. They were subsidizing multinational chemical corporations.[1] The federal dollars only passed through the farmer's checkbook, which served as a conduit between the federal treasury and chemical companies' coffers.

On top of the drought, 1988 brought another challenge. One day while working in our machine shed, we heard banging on the tin roof, like big drops of rain. But it was a bright, sunny day without a cloud in sight. I went outside and looked up, covering the sun with my hand so I wouldn't hurt my eyes. To my amazement, I saw billions and billions of specks dropping out of the sky onto our shed, our farm, everything. Grasshoppers. Before they decimated my crops, I decided to do what I could to try to save the harvest.

I still had a barley field that wasn't organic, so I scrambled to hire a spray plane to douse it with malathion, which immediately kills everything—you're not even supposed to be in the field for twelve hours afterward because you have to wait for the poison to dissipate. Obviously, malathion wasn't an option in my organic wheat field across the creek, so instead I walked around the edge of that field and spread wheat bran coated with *Nosema locustae*, a naturally occurring microbe that is a parasite of grasshoppers. When grasshoppers eat *Nosema locustae*, my friends in the organic community told me, there's a chain effect: the first grasshoppers to ingest the parasite get sick and die, and then their buddies eat them and meet the same fate. Gross, but effective.

Sure enough, in my organic field, the grasshoppers came in from the bordering pasture and ate all around the edge. But then, just as my friends had promised, the plague of insects got sick and died from the *Nosema locustae* as each successive wave of grasshoppers ate their dead, infected brethren. The first fifty feet of my grain was wiped out. But when it came time for harvest, the rest of the field was grasshopper free and I had a fair crop of wheat.

Meanwhile, in the field where I'd sprayed malathion, the grasshoppers were immediately killed—and so was everything else. But within a week or ten days, all their friends came, and by then the poison was gone. Spraying again was out of the question: I was already spending nearly as much on chemical application as my barley was worth, and I didn't want to go further in the hole.

By harvesttime, the crop was greatly reduced in yield and there were grasshoppers everywhere, contaminating the barley and the grain tank of the combine. Not only did I lose most of the field, but I also put considerable money into a chemical that didn't serve its purpose. That was it. I had given my barley field the best that chemical agriculture had to offer. It was not enough. That was the last time I ever applied chemicals to any part of my farm.

Once I transitioned to organic, farming was much more fun. I didn't have to deal with the spray anymore, which was a relief—particularly when the International Agency for Research on Cancer classified our region's most common herbicide as a probable human carcinogen and a California court followed suit by awarding damages to a groundskeeper dying of cancer. And instead of using someone else's canned prescription for my weed problems and my fertility needs, I was designing my own crop rotations, which was the neatest science project ever. Growing my own fertilizer instead of buying it—how cool was that? If you followed some simple principles, like rotating nitrogen-fixing crops with grain crops, you could get pretty good results right away. I had discovered that part in my first year with my organic wheat experiment on alfalfa plowdown. But then the learning never stopped—I kept tinkering with different rotations of crops, different row spacing, different tillage practices, all the while observing my soil and my plants to see what the effects were. My farm became my laboratory.

One of the first things I needed to experiment with was my fertility program—my biological replacement for chemical fertilizer. Some organic farmers, particularly small farmers, replace the fertility of their soil with compost or animal manure. But as a dryland grain farmer with no access to sufficient quantities of either of those things, my best option was to plant leguminous cover crops.

Cover crops are plants that are grown strictly to support the soil rather than to directly produce food or fiber. As their name indicates, these crops literally cover the land, thereby protecting soil from erosion by wind or rain. They replicate this function underground, sending down roots that further prevent erosion by physically holding soil in place. And what's more, cover crop roots don't stop working for the soil when they die: as they continually slough off and decompose, they help build soil organic matter, the living fraction of soil that is the foundation of its fertility and capacity to store water.

In addition, some cover crops are in the bean and pea family (known collectively as legumes), so they can fix nitrogen—which was what I was most interested in as I figured out how to replace chemical fertilizer. Others are prized for their robust root systems, which can improve soil structure or reduce compaction. Blended into untold thousands of different "cocktails" tailored to distinct farming conditions around the world, cover crops are probably the most important tool in the organic farmer's tool kit, and increasingly, non-organic farmers are using them as well. The USDA began funding national surveys on cover crop use in 2011, and within five years, the number of acres that survey respondents planted to cover crops had doubled.[2]

I'd had good success right off the bat with a leguminous cover crop of alfalfa, but most of the early organic farmers in the region were using yellow blossom sweet clover. Although slow to get started, the sweet clover had a two-year growth cycle and was known for producing abundant nitrogen and biomass in its second season. So farmers seeded it right into their grain crop, where it could mature slowly below the canopy of wheat or barley. Protected from weed competition by the canopy cover of the robust grain, the sweet clover could gradually establish itself so that once harvesttime came and the grain was cut, the sweet clover had enough of a head start to really go like gangbusters in year two. Or, at least, that was the theory. But when I tried underseeding sweet clover into my wheat, I found that it wasn't always the underdog it was made out to be. In years when we received extra rainfall, the sweet clover grew so quickly that it came up into my grain, where it stayed all the way through harvest. When the sweet clover went into the combine, the leaves were crushed, releasing a juice that scented my wheat with a distinctive odor. (Don't be fooled by the pleasant-sounding name: if anyone ever offers you a loaf of yellow sweet clover–infused bread, you'll probably want to pass.) But in other years, I had the opposite problem—not *enough* sweet clover. Ironically, this was a problem immediately following years when conditions were just right for the clover—so much so that it spread throughout the ditches and pastures around Big Sandy. This flush of clover would support a big population of sweetclover weevils—troublesome small beetles that chew away at sweet clover leaves in crescent-shaped increments. Then, once the weevils finished their meal in the ditches, they all came to my house the next year and ate up the sweet clover I'd planted for my cover crop.

Frustrated by my boom-and-bust experience with sweet clover, I went back to alfalfa, which worked great for me throughout the early 1990s, when we had a lot of rain. The nitrogen-fixing alfalfa did a brilliant job of growing its own fertility while producing like crazy and crowding out all my weeds.

Then another drought hit us at the end of the decade, and it came to my place a year earlier than it showed up at the neighbors'. My water-loving alfalfa had been sucking moisture from the soil, so I had no reserve. Starved for moisture, my alfalfa didn't germinate properly, leaving two of my fields completely bare. With no cover to shield the soil and no roots to hold it, these fields started blowing away. I was in a world of hurt. I had no soil moisture, which meant I couldn't plant my alfalfa, which meant I couldn't build and protect my soil, which meant I couldn't improve its water-holding capacity, which meant I had no moisture . . . it was a vicious cycle.

So I switched to cover cropping with peas, which had a big seed, so I could plant them deep and reach the little moisture there was farther down. The peas covered the ground effectively and began rebuilding my soil organic matter, but my following wheat crop didn't have as much protein, signaling that it wasn't getting enough nitrogen. Then I started getting new weed problems, and the last straw was when I began noticing root rot in the peas.

Then it dawned on me. I had a solution for managing nutrients and breaking up weed and disease cycles in my cash crop. Rotation. By now, I had several different kinds of wheat in my multiyear crop plan, as well as peas, barley, alfalfa, safflower, and occasionally lentils and flax. If I rotated my cash crops, how come I wasn't rotating my cover crops? So I tried all three of the cover crops I'd tried before: alfalfa, peas, and sweet clover, but this time I rotated them—and I added buckwheat in the mix too. I planned my cover crop rotation in accordance with the conditions of each individual field, to be sure I interrupted any weeds or diseases before they got comfortable, and evened out any nutrient imbalances. I fed the soil what it needed. Then it took care of feeding my plants.

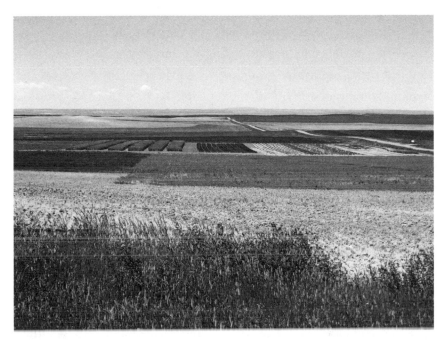

MY FARM IN EARLY SUMMER, WITH COVER CROP FIELDS IN THE FOREGROUND AND TEST PLOTS OF GRAIN AND DRYLAND VEGETABLES JUST BEHIND THEM.
(Photo by Hilary Page)

Granted, I didn't figure all of this out on my own. From the moment I began experimenting on my farm, I had been casting about for colleagues with whom I could compare notes. Since I came from a university background, the first place I looked was Montana State. In 1986, I asked a friend who was a weed scientist at MSU how I could control my weeds without chemicals. He leaned back in his chair and his eyes glazed over. "No one's ever asked me a question like that before," he told me.

That was pretty much the state of things at MSU in the mid-1980s, as it was at nearly all the agricultural universities in the country. The faculties of these institutions had been trained in the same chemical understanding of agriculture that I'd been steeped in at UC Davis, and they didn't understand why a farmer wouldn't want to make use of the latest products developed to help them succeed in the new industrial agribusiness. The dearth of support for research on more ecological approaches to farming was discouraging, but fortunately, I was surrounded by an inquisitive group of free-range scientists in the organic farming community. Many of these people had advanced degrees and had started out on a traditional academic career path before deciding, as I had, that there was no better laboratory than a farm. But whatever level of formal education they had, people in the organic community were tireless experimenters, and they were remarkably generous with their knowledge and experience. It was the spirit of inquiry and cooperation I'd been missing in my lab at Davis—what mattered was the advancement of understanding for the common good, not who landed the biggest grant or made the most money.

One of the most fascinating things we organic farmers learned together was about weeds. In the era of 2,4-D, we'd all gotten used to seeing completely weed-free fields, and these "clean" monocultures became the universally acknowledged sign of a good farmer. Reproducing this vigilantly uniform aesthetic proved difficult to achieve with organic methods, which frustrated a lot of us in the beginning.

But as we diversified our rotations and built up our soils, our weed pressure changed. We had more kinds of weeds, here and there, but none of the large patches of a single pesky plant that we'd always had to contend with when we grew monocultures. As long as we kept an eye on our here-and-there weeds and didn't let them go to seed, our crops crowded them out, and they didn't spread enough to significantly diminish our harvest.

Over time, we found that diverse rotations, sound soil management, and careful monitoring were sufficient to control our weeds so that they never became an economic problem. All we had to do now was change our definition of success, from eradication to management. I decided I could live with seeing a few mustard plants here and there if it meant improving my bottom line and reducing the chemical load on people and the planet.

Of course, my neighbors thought I was completely crazy. They called me the weed farmer. They said organic would never work. They were just waiting to see what would happen first: would I give up or go broke? I got tired of hearing this kind of stuff through the grapevine (nobody said it when I was within earshot), but I didn't want to go down to the coffee shop and argue about it. So I decided to buy a new Caterpillar tractor.

At the time, it was an expensive tractor: sixty or seventy thousand dollars brand-new. Caterpillar was just starting to make tractors that ran on rubber tracks, like a tank, and mine was the first one in the area. I could get in the field two or three days before everybody else because I was on tracks now, and I wasn't going to get stuck in the mud, like you do with wheel tractors. Our farm was right on the highway, so everybody could see. Without saying a word, I think I got the message across: this organic farm is successful.

Then the word out on the street was "Okay, it looks like he can make this work, but it's because he's a PhD." It was the chemical dealers who were pushing this line, which was really quite condescending. Basically, the chemical dealers were telling my neighbors that they weren't smart enough to manage their own fertility and weed control, so they'd better keep buying the dealers' products.

Looking back, I was so naïve. When I first returned home to the farm, I went to one of the nearby weed clinics sponsored by Monsanto (the agricultural chemical and seed giant recently acquired by Bayer), where I made friends with a young chemical rep. We were both chemists by training, just starting our careers, and I figured we had a lot in common. So I asked him if he could help me solve a question I'd been pondering. I knew that herbicides set crops back a little bit—it was well established in the literature that the chemicals stressed out the plants, leading to a small yield reduction. So in a year when there were almost no weeds, it wasn't economical to spray. If you put the plant stress and the cost of the herbicide in the loss column and the weed control benefit in the gain column, the losses outweighed the gain. But I didn't know where the threshold was. So I asked my new friend, "How many weeds do I need to have to make it worthwhile to spray?" I thought it would be very helpful to farmers if Monsanto would do that kind of research on economic thresholds and make it widely available.

The chemical rep listened to me very courteously. "I'll get back to you on that," he said, but of course he never did. Monsanto wasn't interested in economic thresholds. The company just wanted to sell as much chemical as possible. It's not a win-win mentality for them. If the farmer wins, fine, but if he loses and goes out of business, Monsanto still gets its money and there will be another guy to take over the farm and keep buying products. So the company pushes its products very hard, and it tries to discredit anybody who questions it. As the organic movement began to gain steam in the late 1980s and early 1990s, agricultural chemical companies responded with vigorous attacks on the credibility of organic practices, as well as on individual organic researchers and advocates. These "information campaigns," as the chemical industry called them, targeted nearly every major rural institution farmers trusted: banks, ag publications, and the major farm organizations.

One day in the early 1990s, the ag lender at my local bank told me about a letter he had received from the area chemical rep. "If any of your customers are proposing to abandon the proven methods of modern agriculture for the high-risk niche of organic production," the chemical rep had written to the banker, "we hope you will not support such a change by lending money to such an ill-conceived enterprise."

Meanwhile, farm publications were reminded of the substantial advertising dollars flowing from the chemical industry and were encouraged to limit the exposure of organic successes. I remember an article about my farm that ran in one of those magazines in the early 1990s. The reporter went into great detail about the diversity of my crops, my rotations, and my direct marketing efforts. But there was not one mention of the word "organic."

The primary targets of the chemical industry's information campaign, however, were the major national farm organizations. By sponsoring their conventions, the chemical companies infused them with their talking points, which filtered down from national meetings to local chapters, where organic farmers like me were ridiculed as fools.

Nobody said anything negative to my face, though, because when I showed up at Farm Bureau meetings, I was there with the state president—my dad. He was held in very high esteem in the agribusiness community, not just in the state but at the national level too. So people just kind of shook their heads at me and figured I'd been in California too long.

Then I got more involved in the Farm Bureau myself and was appointed to the national wheat committee. I was having so much success with organic methods, I figured I should share the good news, so I started telling all these Farm Bureau wheat growers about it. At first, everybody's eyebrows went up because mostly they'd heard this only from hippies on two-acre farms. Not the son of the Montana Farm Bureau president who'd handed out cookies for Goldwater as a kid and was now farming 2,400 acres of prime wheat ground. No one believed it. I was on this committee for three years, though, and by the end, some of my fellow committee members started coming up to me—not in public, but in private—wanting to learn more about organic.

One reason my neighbors were getting more and more interested in organic farming was that the market was taking off. I sold my first load of organically grown wheat in 1984. By 1988, organic accounted for half my business at Montana Flour and Grains. By 1992, it *was* the business: 98 percent of sales were organic. By then, I was philosophically committed too, but it wasn't only my beliefs that drove my transition; it was also my customers. To my astonishment, my dad was more bullish about this new marketing opportunity than I was.

In 1986, when I was still in the midst of my first organic experiment, a TV reporter came to interview me. This was before I'd even harvested my first organic crop, and I was really early on in my learning process. After a few fairly innocuous questions, I figured things were going along just fine. But then the reporter hit me with a stunner out of left field. "Tell me, now," she asked, "you're selling organic. But is organic really better for you?"

No one had ever asked me that question. I was converting to organic because I thought it was a better way to *farm*. The economics were better for me, and I thought it was more fun and made more sense. Meanwhile, I'd started selling organic wheat to bakers in Southern California because that's what the bakers wanted. I didn't have to explain to them why it was better to *eat*; they had already decided it was better, for taste or nutrition or the environment or whatever, and that's why they were coming to me and asking for it. So I was more focused on the "how" of organic than the "why" at that time. I kind of stumbled all over the reporter's question, and finally she said, "Well, maybe I should ask that in a different way."

I came home and told my dad that I'd been asked point-blank if organic was better for you, thinking he would join me in a good laugh about my being caught off guard by such a left-field question. But that wasn't his response at all. "I hope you didn't muff the ball on that one," my dad said, a serious look on his face.

I was flabbergasted. Dad had just given me the green light to convert the farm to organic. You might think the sixty-six-year-old former Montana Farm Bureau president—the first farmer in our area to adopt chemical fertilizers—would have needed an adjustment period to warm up to the new farming system. But instead, he was actually disappointed that I hadn't prepared myself to proclaim the benefits of organically grown food, given that this was my market and the future of our farm. I don't think he ever saw organics as the future of global agriculture, the way I do now, but in terms of the economic future of our family farm, he saw it immediately.

My dad passed away four years ago, just before his ninety-fourth birthday, so he was around to see my whole trajectory in organic as I rapidly became quite a vocal advocate. Never once did he try to defend farm chemicals as some time-honored tradition. The truth was, he'd started using them only fairly recently, since they hadn't been available when he was young. Chemical farming was merely one approach my dad experimented with to try to solve a problem. It wasn't at all difficult for him to accept that these chemicals were not the answer to everything and that I might have found a better solution. To him, organic farming was much like the TV he bought in 1954, which was one of the first in our neighborhood. Another innovation.

For me, though, organic farming was more than an innovation. It was a 180-degree shift in the character of agriculture: from an extractive activity that mined the value of the soil to a regenerative activity that could sustain that value for millennia. With a healthy soil, all sorts of other problems that farmers complained about were averted in the root zone: weeds, disease, and fertility problems were resolved before they got started, at a fraction of the cost necessary to fight them down the road with chemicals. Looking beyond my own farm community, I saw that this regenerative means of producing food could shift the fate of humanity on this earth, from continued degradation of our life-support services to responsible citizenship in the ecological community. If there was a way to eliminate world hunger, decrease chronic disease, and live peacefully together on the planet, this transformation in our agriculture seemed to me a critical piece of that puzzle. Combining a repertoire of time-tested practices—like cover cropping and crop rotation—with some of the best science of my generation, I saw that organic farmers were already making strides toward that future.

Going organic taught me many lessons that have served me well in business: tackle problems at their root, work *with* nature rather than against it, and don't dump so much capital into gross gains that you end up with net losses. What began as a simple attempt to serve a customer became an eye-opening realization: using organic methods, we could add back so much value to the 52 percent of US land that is in agriculture.[3] Managed correctly, farms not only can be more profitable but also can produce more nutritious food and sustain healthy soils—while storing atmospheric carbon, maintaining healthy watersheds, and providing critical habitat for pollinators. In the era of climate change, we need to think more and more about how to add this kind of ecological value to everything we do in business. We don't have a planet B.

When I started selling my own wheat, whole, I recovered the economic value I'd previously lost to industrial processors. When I started farming it organically, I also began recovering the ecological value I'd lost to industrial production—and to chemical companies, which had been cutting my net profits to nearly zero. But in order to fully restore the value of this grain, I needed to follow it all the way back to its source: the seed. I hadn't thought much about the varieties of wheat I was planting beyond their yield and protein potential—typically I went with what seeds worked best on our own farm or what the nearby experiment station recommended. But a chance encounter with a friend who had a rare health condition was about to change all that.

CHAPTER 5:

King Tut's Wheat

Not long after I started selling *organic* wheat, one of my customers asked for *stone-ground* wheat. Flour.

My first response was that I didn't know anything about milling. I told the customer I wasn't in the milling business. I tried to talk him into installing the mill at his bakery so he'd have the flour freshly ground, on demand. But he said that was too much of a hassle. He was interested in buying finished flour. When I figured out how to make it, I should call him back.

My cousin did some research and found a company just north of us, in British Columbia, that was importing stone mills from Austria. They had a beautiful little model available for just six or seven thousand dollars, which was within my budget. The salesman said it was foolproof: all I had to do was plug it into the wall.

When the mill arrived, I quickly discovered that the plug wasn't compatible with my American power outlet; so much for plug and play! The necessary adapter was easy enough to obtain at the hardware store, but as I peered into the nooks and crannies of the unfamiliar machine, I realized I had a bigger problem: I had no idea how to use it. Following an initial wave of disappointment, I had an aha moment. What a ridiculous expectation, that a grain mill would essentially do its job automatically with no input from me. This was the commodity mindset: standardize everything so it can be done industrially. The stone mill was telling me to walk away from that expectation, toward craft, care—and higher-value flour.

I called up a friend in Great Falls who was selling insurance and hated his job. "Why don't you move up to Fort Benton and become a miller?" I propositioned him. I think his wife took a little convincing, but they made the leap. Within weeks, he was up in Fort Benton constructing a mill room for the building we had just rented. Once that was finished, my new miller headed off to Ohio and Pennsylvania to study with experienced masters willing to share their craft. These master millers taught my friend the tools of the trade: How close to place the two millstones, depending on the desired texture of the flour. How to read that texture to recognize when the stones were smoothing away their grinding face. And how to sharpen or "dress" the stones, chiseling the signature pattern that turned grain into flour, while providing ventilation to ensure the proper temperature for the process. This last point was critical: if the temperature within the mill got too high, it could destroy some of the nutrients in the flour. The longtime millers in Ohio and Pennsylvania were sticklers on this matter. You had to carefully control the rate at which grain flowed through the machine, or you would cook the life right out of it.

After taking in all this wisdom, my friend came back to Montana a bona fide miller, adding stone-ground flour to the repertoire of our steadily growing business. We were no longer just Montana Wheat Company; now we were Montana Flour and Grains.

I don't remember whether any TV reporters came by to ask whether stone-ground flour was better than its conventionally milled counterpart. But if they had, I would have known the answer this time. With stone-ground whole wheat flour, you get 100 percent of what's in the wheat, in the original proportions nature intended. Conventional whole wheat mills did things differently. They separated the grain with a roller mill, as they normally did for white flour, and then they added back some bran and germ to make the "whole wheat" product look earthier. US Food and Drug Administration standards for products labeled "whole wheat" stated that all three components of the grain had to be present in their original proportions, but the agency did nothing to verify that the standard was being met. Investigative journalism would later reveal what rumors were already indicating: in order to preserve shelf life, conventional whole wheat mills often threw out the oily germ.[1] So if you wanted real-deal whole wheat, you had to get stone-ground.

My cousin and I were pretty pleased when we called our customer back and told him we had his stone-ground whole wheat flour. We asked him how much he wanted on his next order. "That's fantastic," the customer said, "I'll take a thousand pounds." A thousand pounds? I wondered if I'd heard him wrong. A thousand pounds was hardly enough to pay our light bill.

We'd invested all this money into renting a plant, converting it to a milling room, buying a mill, building a ramp to load pallets onto delivery trucks, buying a forklift, and hiring a full-time employee to run the whole thing. The payoff was a high-value product, but while we waited to find someone to buy a little more of it, all this overhead was eating up most of the profits from our grain sales. We needed to sell some flour. And soon.

In 1986, we rented a booth at Natural Products Expo West in Anaheim, California, one of the largest natural food trade shows in the world. My parents came along to help. I had one goal, which was to find buyers for our stone-ground whole grain flour. But my dad decided to bring a jar of "King Tut's wheat"—the same stuff I'd seen at the Fort Benton County Fair some two decades earlier.

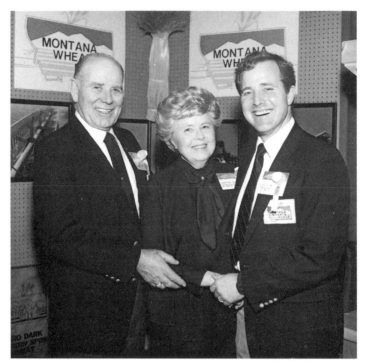

WITH MY PARENTS, MAKING OUR FIRST NATURAL FOODS SHOW
APPEARANCE IN ANAHEIM, CALIFORNIA, 1986.
(Photo courtesy of Bob Quinn)

I'd tried to make a go of marketing the novelty wheat myself, back when I was finishing graduate school at UC Davis and casting about for projects to supplement my income and support my growing family. One day during my graduate studies, I was idly walking down the corridor of Briggs Hall, a new building constructed to accommodate the growing number of students and faculty in the biological sciences. In case you're picturing an idyllic academic setting from a movie like *Love Story*— bright, charming brick building amid greenery—let me assure you, the place looks more like a fortress from some science fiction film—or a prison. To make matters worse, I was working in the basement of this concrete homage to brutalist architecture. At least we had windows.

Anyway, I needed a break, so I walked down the hall and got a package of Corn Nuts from the vending machine. To stall a few more moments before returning to my lab, I read the label on the back and spotted the words "Made with a giant corn." Fascinating, I thought, recalling the man who had wowed me at the Fort Benton County Fair with his novelty grain. I wonder if these guys would be interested in a giant wheat.

Forgetting my dissertation for the moment, I called up the Corn Nuts company, encouraged that it was nearby, in Oakland. The person I spoke to put me in touch with a product development specialist, and he turned out to be a fellow member of Alpha Gamma Rho, the agriculturally focused fraternity I'd joined as an undergraduate at Montana State. This fellow had gone to Oregon State, but his name sounded familiar, and after a few moments on the phone together we realized we'd met at a leadership conference the fraternity had sponsored in Bozeman. I heartened to discover that I knew the guy, I told him the whole story about the wheat I'd seen at the county fair a decade earlier. "Sounds interesting," he said. "Send some over."

More than a little excited, I immediately phoned my dad and asked if he could find me some seed. Dad hunted around town, and after a few days, he located a friend in Fort Benton, Sparky Sparks, who had a jar in his basement. We took a couple of tablespoons of that seed and sent it to my friend at Corn Nuts. "This stuff is fantastic," he gushed. "It makes a wonderful snack. I'll take ten thousand pounds."

"Uh, we don't quite have ten thousand pounds," I told the product development guy. I didn't tell him we barely had *one* pound. "But give us a couple years and we'll get you all you need." I called up my dad again and told him to plant the rest of the seed in the garden. Dad planted it, harvested it, shelled it out by hand, and planted it again. When he harvested that second crop, we contracted with a seed company in California to grow it out over the winter. Within a year and a half, we had fifty pounds.

I got back in touch with Corn Nuts, eager to share the good news. But my friend was gone. Nobody had his contact information, and his successors weren't interested in our giant wheat. My dad took the fifty pounds of the seed we'd so meticulously grown out and put it in the shed. There it sat for half a decade—until he decided to take a jar of it to this food show.

After three days at Expo West, my cousin and I both had pockets full of referrals and business cards. We were thrilled.

My dad had shown the King Tut's wheat to everybody who walked by, which must have been thousands of people, but he had just one prospect. And yet, the guy followed through. The first customer for our ancient wheat was a fellow named Carlos Richardson, who had just started a macrobiotic food store in San Diego with his wife. He said he'd buy all we could grow.

Taking Carlos at his word, we planted all fifty pounds of the ancient wheat, on half an acre. An agronomist from the Montana State experiment station in Havre came down with their little plot combine to help us cut it, so we wouldn't unintentionally mix it with any of the modern wheat that might be in our big combine. From that half acre, we got enough seed to plant twenty acres the following year, and from those twenty acres we had enough to plant eighty acres our third year. Now we had enough to supply the market, and we were ready to sell it. And unlike the Corn Nuts product development team, Carlos was still eager to buy it.

I figured this ancient wheat could be a good novelty crop for us on a few acres. A small but not insignificant little sideshow to the flour mill. So I contacted one of the customers who was buying my ordinary wheat, Bob Anderson from Health Best in Escondido, California. I thought Bob might be interested in a few pounds of the ancient grain, for bulk bins or something. But as soon as he heard my story, he had bigger ideas. I sent him a sample, and Bob took our giant wheat to Royal Angelus Macaroni Company, which was trying to develop a more palatable whole wheat pasta.

In the mid-1980s, whole wheat pasta was pretty terrible. Gritty. Grainy. Bitter. It scratched the back of your throat. The reason for this was that modern varieties of wheat had been bred to produce extremely hard bran—the fibrous part of the grain that formed its outer coating—so that it would be easy for roller mills to flake it off. The assumption was that the wheat was going to be refined and eaten as white flour, white bread, Twinkies, mac and cheese from a box—the staples of the contemporary American diet. The bran wasn't bred to be nutty or flavorful or nutritious; it was bred to be readily discarded.[2]

When people started getting concerned about the nutritional value they were losing by flaking off the bran, they tried to put it back. That was the idea with conventional "whole wheat," as opposed to stone milling. Go ahead and refine away the bran and the germ and then try to put some of it back later. But when you put the bran back later, the sum of the parts never did equal the whole, nutritionally speaking.[3] And unless you really pulverized that bran, you had a texture problem. It was hard as a rock and splintered like glass.

Royal Angelus wanted to make whole wheat pasta more appetizing, so they were trying all sorts of different experiments to fix the texture. Bob Anderson figured they might want to give our ancient wheat a try, so he took a sample over to their headquarters and made his pitch. "Thanks, but we're not interested," the owner told him, and Bob figured that was that. But as he walked out the door and back to his car, he found himself being chased down by Santo Zito, the Sicilian-born artisan who ran Royal Angelus's test kitchen and managed pasta production. Santo knew about ancient wheat from his relatives in Sicily, who'd given him seeds from older varieties that looked similar to the ones we were growing. "Let's give it a try," he told Bob, taking the sample back to his kitchen.

Over the course of the next week, Santo transformed the grain into pasta, grinding it into flour and then experimenting with just the right ratio of water and flour to create the perfect dough. When he cooked up his initial batch of ancient wheat macaroni, the first thing that struck him was the pungent aroma that filled the room. But even more remarkable was the consistency of the pasta when he put it in his mouth. It was smooth. Almost silky.

When Santo thought about it, it wasn't hard to understand why. Here was a wheat that preceded all the aggressive breeding for hard bran. It was *meant* to be eaten whole.

Once Santo gave his boss a taste of the new ancient wheat pasta, Royal Angelus promptly introduced it into the product line. Santo gave me a box full of samples, which I shared with a number of my neighbors. My dad took some too, and he gave it to a good friend of ours, Laura, who had very severe environmental sensitivities.

When I say "severe": Laura came to church one time when we had a new building, and she had to leave because of the formaldehyde fumes emanating from the new carpet. She couldn't tolerate chemicals at all. Her muscles would stop working, and if it got bad enough, she would collapse. She couldn't be around anyone wearing perfume or cologne. And she had to be very careful about what she ate.

I wouldn't have had the audacity to give this woman any kind of food. But my farm was organic by then, so I guess my dad thought she might appreciate a box of pasta made from wheat that was grown without the use of chemicals. Laura thought it was worth trying, so she decided to take a chance on it. The next day, she called my parents' house and asked my dad, "What is this stuff? It makes me feel better."

It was still more than a decade before I would meet a team of researchers in Italy who would make groundbreaking discoveries about the effects of an ancient grain diet on chronic disease. Still more than a decade before I'd meet the man who would tell me he'd been in declining health, with ailments that stumped his doctors and threatened his life, before switching to ancient wheat and making a full recovery. Still more than a decade before I would receive the phone call from a mother, crying, thanking me for growing the only grain her daughter could eat.

But that conversation with Laura in the late 1980s was my wake-up call that growing wheat organically and leaving the grain whole wasn't enough to recover the full value of this staple food. The most insidious way in which the staff of life had been devalued involved transformations to the seed itself, when industry breeders sacrificed all else to focus on marginal gains in yield and loaf volume. I had stumbled onto ancient wheat by chance and had initially seen it as a fun novelty crop with an intriguing legend. But Laura's epiphany led me on a long search to understand how heritage grains—the varieties our forefarmers selected and saved—can help us recover what we've lost.

CHAPTER 6:

Growing Partners

Big agribusiness is all about trade secrets. Their idea of success is developing a valuable product and then controlling it as tightly as possible. I think the more rewarding approach is to share it. In the case of our organically raised ancient whole wheat, I was coming to understand that sharing it as broadly as possible could help solve some financial troubles for farmers and some serious environmental problems on thousands of acres of farmland. I was just getting an inkling, after my friend Laura's experience, of what it might mean for people's health. But sharing the grain was also beneficial to my business. Rather than trying to control everything myself, I recruited a network of partners to help me—a network that now numbers in the thousands.

But first, we had to figure out what to call this ancient wheat. In the early days, we just called it "King Tut's wheat," like the man had at the Fort Benton County Fair. We tried a few variations on that. But if this grain was really from ancient Egypt, I thought, we ought to find out what the ancient Egyptians called it.

In 1988, I drove down to the Great Falls Library and picked up *An Egyptian Hieroglyphic Dictionary* by E. A. Wallis Budge. To my delight,

Budge had included an entry for wheat, and it included a transliteration of the ancient Egyptian character: kamut. The dictionary wasn't terribly clear on pronunciation, but I didn't think people would line up to buy kuh-MUTT pasta. So we called it kuh-MOOT.

Then I had a bit of a dilemma. My dad told me we needed to trademark it. I hadn't considered that at first, given my philosophy about sharing a good thing, but Dad told me that if we had any success with this, other people might try to sell lower-quality wheat under the same name. This is exactly what happened with spelt—industry scientists looking for yield gains began crossbreeding ancient grain with modern wheat and calling it spelt, to the dismay of people with wheat sensitivities who thought they were eating something they could comfortably digest.[1] This cautionary tale convinced me of the need for a consumer protection mechanism for our ancient wheat that would function as a legally binding guarantee. So I told Dad to go ahead and draw up the paperwork for a trademark.

Our trademark was concerning to many of my friends in the organic community, who were watching the conventional seed industry assert ever more ownership over the basic building blocks of life. After ten thousand years of farmers saving their own seed and replanting it, expanding biotechnology companies like Monsanto were taking advantage of a 1980 US Supreme Court decision, *Diamond v. Chakrabarty*, that allowed them to apply for utility patents on their varieties. Even though most of the genetic material in Monsanto seeds had been developed by farmers over hundreds of generations, the corporation could make a few small modifications and then patent the whole package (and potentially its genetic components as well)—meaning farmers could be sued for planting it without buying Monsanto's license. Rightfully so, many farmers were irate, and they were suspicious of anything that looked like an attempt to claim ownership rights over seed.

A trademark is very different from a patent, I explained to my friends. I had no interest in owning the variety of wheat that we were selling under the brand name Kamut. My belief was, and still is, that this wheat is a gift from God, and it's not for any one person to own. Any farmer should be able to plant it, save the seed, and either consume it or sell it to someone else. This ancient wheat has a generic name, which we would later learn is khorasan. Many people now grow and sell khorasan wheat, and I think they should be able to do so freely.

But if they want to sell it under the brand name Kamut, they have to go through our verification protocol—because the Kamut trademark means more than khorasan wheat. I wrote into the legal definition that it has to be grown organically and it can't be hybridized or adulterated with modern wheat, which some people have trouble digesting (for reasons I would come to understand later). That's my guarantee to the customer: no chemicals have been used to grow this wheat, and it hasn't been hybridized or adulterated, so no genetic value has been subtracted from it along the way. It's the real thing.

The next question, of course, was what to actually make out of this grain. I knew I didn't want to get into the food-manufacturing business. The whole ordeal of graduating from stored grain to flour had been quite enough, and in the early days of the Kamut project, we still hadn't quite gotten out from under all the capital expenses and overhead associated with the mill and the grain-cleaning plant we had added to it in 1989. My cousin had sold off his business in 1988 and moved on to other pursuits, and as a one-man show as far as capital outlays were concerned, I was wary of biting off more than I could chew. So my philosophy from that point forward was to focus on what I did best—production—and find partners whose talent shined in the test kitchen. I called them partners, not customers, because I found that a more accurate description. I could only succeed if my partners succeeded too, so if they had problems, I tried to troubleshoot them. I tried to put a little more grain in the bag than was on the label, and if it didn't work in someone's product, I took it back, no questions asked.

Our dream partner was Arrowhead Mills, the cereal company that epitomized success in organic grain in those days. The company's founder and board chair, Frank Ford, was one of the organic industry's most prominent advocates and a celebrity of sorts on the natural food show circuit. A big man with a firm handshake, Frank strolled the show floor as though he were its mayor, greeting everyone by name and projecting an infectious confidence. When I first introduced myself to him in 1986, with my business still in its infancy, Frank slapped me on the back and gestured jovially to the president of his company. "Come on over here," he told him, "and meet our new competition."

For the next five years, whenever we went to a food show, we religiously stopped by the Arrowhead Mills booth with whatever samples my mother had cooked up: Kamut shortbread, Kamut pasta salad, Kamut cookies. Finally, Arrowhead's product development people came over to our booth and started asking us questions about the grain. In 1991, they decided to have a go at making a cereal out of it. It was called Kamut Flakes, and within six months of its release, it was their number two seller.

Kamut Flakes caused a huge jump in our growth: we were doubling our sales every year. Just as I'd found with my first business venture, doubling your sales doesn't look very impressive in the beginning, when you're starting from nothing. But after a couple of years, the numbers started to add up. Other cereal companies jumped on board. There was a puff product made with honey that really should have been in the candy section instead of the cereal section. One of my favorites was a thinly rolled and toasted flake—sort of a Wheaties knock-off—which had very few added ingredients and really highlighted the unique taste of the grain. Then Nature's Path started making a heritage cereal line

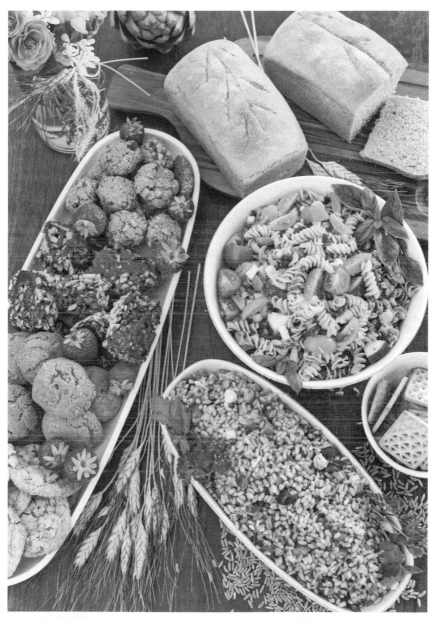

AN ANCIENT GRAIN PICNIC: KAMUT PASTA SALAD, WHOLE GRAIN KAMUT
SALAD, KAMUT BREAD, AND AN ASSORTMENT OF KAMUT COOKIES.
(Photo by Gerald Freyer)

incorporating Kamut grain, which has done very well: they're now our largest customer in North America.

It didn't stop at cereal and pasta. There was pancake mix. Bread. Frozen entrée pasta. One company wanted to make a green drink with it, like a wheatgrass drink.

As our business grew, I insisted on a pricing philosophy that flabbergasted some of the larger companies that came calling: I wouldn't give them a volume discount. I didn't think smaller companies should have a disadvantage in the marketplace just because they were small, and I didn't think we should be playing games with our prices. The price of the grain should reflect its value, plain and simple. Our business model wasn't based on trying to cut corners and find shortcut economies of scale—it was based on providing the same quality at large volumes that we would with a small batch—and vice versa. That policy might have cost me a few business deals, but on the other hand, I think it helped me find partners who shared my philosophy—of whom, I was pleased to discover, there seemed to be no shortage.

With all these partners making Kamut cereal and pasta and pancake mix, demand had long since begun to outstrip the volume I could supply from my farm. I could have bought more land, but I was more interested in sharing the benefits of growing high-value organic crops with other farmers. Now that I'd grown a network of partners on the manufacturing side of the business, it was time to do the same for production.

In 1987, I had helped found Montana's first chapter of the Organic Crop Improvement Association, a nonprofit organic certifier, and I became the association's first president. We had the initial meeting around my kitchen table. Because of my experience helping those first OCIA farms with their certification, I was familiar with their practices, so I started asking some of those growers if they wanted to grow a little Kamut grain and sell it to our mill.

"What's the yield like on this Kamut wheat?" asked one of these growers, an understated guy named Randy Hinebauch, who had started converting his farm to organic the same year I did. I told Randy we didn't have enough experience with the grain to say for sure what its yield potential was, but it was a good bit lower than the varieties he was used to seeding.

"Is there some kind of premium on that, for protein or something?" Randy asked, trying to figure out how ancient grain could pencil out as a sound business decision. I told him that the grain did indeed have premium value, and that we could pay him at least double the price per bushel he was getting on his typical organic wheat, with an advance contract and prompt payment upon delivery. Never one to rush into a decision, Randy thought about it, then asked me some questions about how the ancient wheat fit into a crop rotation and what sort of management it needed. "Well, Bob, it sure sounds like we could come out ahead on this, compared to the modern wheat," Randy surmised. "I'll try it."

Not wanting to lead farmers down the primrose path, I investigated the best growing conditions for the ancient grain. It always did well on my farm, but I noticed disease problems in regions with higher levels of rainfall. After arranging for a network of experimental test plots in wheat-growing areas all over the world, I eventually arrived at a rule of thumb—anywhere that got enough rain to grow a good crop of corn was too wet for a healthy Kamut crop. The ancient grain did best in semi-arid, non-irrigated conditions—exactly what we have a lot of in north central Montana.

Since it was an ancient variety that hadn't been bred to increase yield potential, Kamut grain was lower yielding than the commodity wheat that farmers—even organic farmers—typically planted. But it was higher value. People were willing to pay more for it because of its flavor and nutritional benefits (which, again, I would learn much more about later). So I decided to set the price at three times the current value of conventional wheat and keep it stable, unlike the year-to-year roller coaster of the commodity wheat market. I wanted to be sure the farmers got a fair deal that they could count on.

Pretty soon, I realized I'd gone a little overboard: the contracts were so lucrative that some farmers wanted to grow nothing but our ancient wheat! This completely defeated the point of encouraging farmers to plant healthy organic rotations. Ancient or not, any variety of wheat grown year after year will draw down the soil's nitrogen and organic matter and lead to pest and disease problems. So we made a rule that farmers couldn't grow Kamut grain on more than 20 percent of their cultivated acreage, and we required that they grow a leguminous cover crop the year before the ancient wheat. From then on, we've explained to growers that our premium is designed to support the soil-building practices that support their farms—which, in turn, support them. We want to add value not just to the crop they sell this year, to us. We want to add value to their land, which we hope will support their family for generations. In the meantime, we want to help them weather the challenges they face now, like drought, weeds, and disease.

Along with most commodity crops—corn, soybeans, cotton—modern wheat has been bred to maximize yields under ideal conditions. Put it in just the right soil, with just the right amount of water, a perfect balance of nutrients, ideal temperature, and no adverse weather—and voilà, you've got sixty to eighty bushels per acre.

You don't have to be a farmer to recognize that this is not generally how real life goes. Real life involves cold snaps and hailstorms and insect pests. In real life, not everybody has center pivot irrigation to make the rain fall artificially when it's not coming out of the sky. And on a Montana wheat farm, real life inevitably involves drought.

Like many ancient grains selected by real-life farmers under real-life conditions over hundreds of generations, Kamut plants are drought resistant. If you look at a graph of average yields under different amounts of annual rainfall, modern wheat has a clear yield advantage over our ancient wheat at about thirteen or fourteen inches, our typical yearly moisture in Big Sandy. But as rainfall decreases, Kamut yields drop more slowly than modern wheat yields, narrowing the gap between the two trend lines. Once it gets dry enough that modern wheat yields sink below ten bushels per acre, our ancient wheat actually starts to outyield the modern wheat. And as it keeps getting dryer, modern wheat yields will eventually go to zero. The Kamut plants hang on. Very rarely do their yields go to zero. These are not the kinds of tests plant breeders performed on wheat varieties when I was in graduate school, when the objective was to maximize yields under ideal conditions. But in our warming world, these kinds of "what if" scenarios are becoming increasingly important.

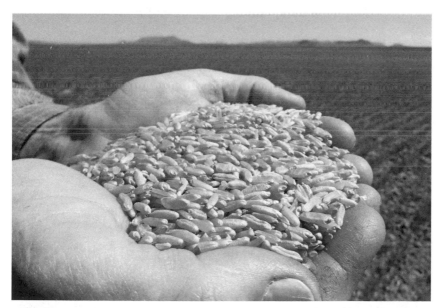

STANDING IN A KAMUT FIELD IN LATE SPRING, HOLDING LAST YEAR'S GRAIN IN MY HANDS.
(Photo by Hilary Page)

Besides drought, another problem that really exasperates wheat farmers in our area is damage from sawflies. Sawflies lay their eggs in the stems of wheat plants, so when the little sawfly babies hatch into worms, they crawl down the stem, eating all the way. When the immature sawflies get to the bottom of the plant, they build a cocoon and cut a ring around the wheat stem right above it, so as to have an easy escape route when they emerge later, as a fly. This incision in the wheat stem isn't a big problem when the plant is still green. But as the crop ripens in the summer, the stem dries out and becomes brittle. For the desiccated stalk, the sawfly damage is like a perforation—as soon as a gust of wind hits, the top of the plant snaps off and falls to the ground. If things get to that stage, it's a total loss for the farmer.

To hedge against sawfly damage, some farmers swathe their grain before it ripens, as you would with hay, or as we used to do with oats when I was a kid. A swather is a machine that will lay the grain on the ground in neat rows, where it can finish ripening and dry out until the farmer comes by and picks it up with a combine. This saves the grain from falling over, but swathing comes with its own risks. Not only does it double the time and fuel spent on harvest to run the extra machine through the field—it also means you've got most of your annual income sitting out there in the field in windrows on the ground, tempting rain, hail, and windstorms.

So when growers select which wheat variety to plant, they pay a lot of attention to its sawfly resistance. Plant breeders who work with modern wheat have tried hard to get this trait into the mix, along with the non-negotiable priorities of agribusiness: high yield, high protein, and high loaf volume. They've had varying degrees of success. But our Kamut growers seldom have problems with sawflies: the stems of these ancient wheat plants are so thick that the troublesome insects have trouble penetrating them.

That's not to say our growers haven't had any problems. They like that Kamut plants are resistant to drought and sawflies, but for people who are used to growing commodity wheat with chemicals, growing an ancient grain, organically, means a steep learning curve. And while the attitude about organics at our land grant universities and experiment stations has improved considerably since my first visit with my weed scientist friend at Montana State over thirty years ago, there are still very few resources dedicated to helping organic growers with their day-to-day questions about operations.

So as our grower network started to approach triple digits, we decided to hire a full-time field person—essentially an extension agent for Kamut farmers. Our field person focuses on three things: helping new organic growers get started, helping our experienced growers who are having a specific problem, and monitoring across the grower network to see what practices are producing the best crops. On any given day, he might be helping a transitioning grower figure out how to fill out organic certification paperwork and design a balanced crop rotation. Or helping an experienced grower identify pesticide drift from a neighboring farm and seek recourse. Or monitoring whether ancient wheat planted after alfalfa did better than ancient wheat planted after peas.

The other thing we do to try to add value for our farmers is supply them with high-quality seed. We select the best seed from the previous year's crop, across our entire grower network. We test it for purity and vigor and make sure it will germinate well. We run it through our cleaning equipment to be sure it's not mixed with modern wheat or barley or anything else. And then we provide it to growers free of cost—all we ask is that they replace it at harvesttime. By essentially sharing our seed-saving operation among more than one hundred farms, we're able to reduce expenses for farmers and improve everyone's chances of success.

Not to harp on it too much, but this is not the direction things are going with seeds for mainstream agribusiness. A staggering 92 percent of corn and 94 percent of soy is now genetically engineered, using proprietary genetics.[2] That means farmers can't even save their own seed: they have to buy new seed every year from Monsanto at exorbitantly high prices. I have some corn farmer friends in the Midwest who want non–genetically modified seed and are having trouble finding it. That's how aggressively these companies have cornered the market. There is some non-GMO seed out there, and that's what organic farmers are required to use, but the majority of the plant-breeding resources have shifted to biotech because that's where the big money is being made. As funding dwindles for public plant-breeding programs at universities, the university researchers who are left are increasingly looking to industry partners to fund their work, which means focusing on industry priorities: lucrative biotech varieties. Meanwhile, as university jobs become scarcer, an increasing share of plant breeders go to work directly for Monsanto, Syngenta, or another seed industry giant, so they aren't accountable to the public interest at all. What all this means is that only a handful of breeders is left to work on non-GMO varieties. No matter how hard they try, it's impossible for this small group of scientists to ensure that all farmers across the country have access to high-quality non-GMO seed adapted to their area and suitable for their conditions. This lack of capacity in non-GMO plant breeding plays right into Monsanto's hands—the company has been frighteningly aggressive in its strategic moves to stamp out any value in the food system that doesn't flow through its own intellectual property. This doesn't stop at GMOs either: the biotech firms have recently reinvested in research and development of hybrid wheat seeds[3] (which, like GMOs, have to be bought each year rather than saved) and are working to lock up the parent strains of these hybrids as "trade secrets" so that public breeders can't access them.

My business model is just the opposite: I think we should be adding value all along the supply chain rather than trying to concentrate it in the middle. To my mind, there's a fatal flaw in economic thinking that measures the success of a business by its ability to amass a lot of capital and control in the hands of a single entity. I measure the success of my business by the degree to which it's added economic, ecological, and nutritional value all along the supply chain: For the hundreds of independent owner-operators who now farm Kamut grain on thousands of acres of certified organic cropland. For the over 3,500 artisans who make it into pasta, cereal, bread, or another food. My job is to make sure everyone in the network gets a fair price and has the opportunity to succeed—they, in turn, ensure the integrity of the product. Instead of fighting over pieces of a small pie, we share a great big one. Since we're not forking over huge chunks of the pie to a handful of multinationals, there's plenty to go around.

Fortunately for wheat growers, our crop hasn't gone the GMO route yet. Not for lack of trying on the part of Monsanto. It is chomping at the bit to get wheat country on its program, and it even put some test plots in Montana in 2002 and 2003.[4] Some wheat farmers welcomed this research, believing it might benefit them. But so far, GMO wheat has been stymied because our markets for commodity wheat from the American prairie—principally in Asia—don't want it. No sense growing something you can't sell.

International markets were the furthest thing from my mind as we were launching the Kamut project in the early 1990s. California was exotic enough for me. And my real focus was on building a regional economy and seeing if I could slow the hemorrhaging of the population in places like Big Sandy.

But one day, I was sitting at the kitchen table with my dad when the phone rang. I was busy with something, so Dad picked up the phone. "Oh no, we're not interested in shipping anything to Europe," I heard him saying.

"Who was that?" I asked.

"Oh, some outfit called Lima," Dad replied offhandedly.

I was still pretty green, but I'd been to a few food shows by then and gotten to know the organic scene from my work with the Organic Crop Improvement Association. I knew Lima wasn't just any old outfit.

"Dad, they're one of the leading organic companies in Europe," I said, surprised and aghast at the same time. My face fell as I realized we'd just snubbed one of the most respected distributors of whole grain, macrobiotic food. Dad was unmoved.

"We can't be shipping this stuff overseas," he said. "We don't know anything about that."

If I'd been in a jocular frame of mind, it would have been humorous. Here was my dad—the guy who'd gotten the first TV in the neighborhood, the guy who'd brought our ancient grain to a California food show in the first place, the guy who'd admonished me for missing an opportunity to promote organics when the local reporter had come out a few years ago—passing up a new opportunity. Meanwhile, here I was—the guy who'd never envisioned planting Kamut seed on more than twenty acres or so, who'd told people it was probably good only for pasta, for heaven's sake—trying to talk him into it. The tables had certainly turned!

But I wasn't in a jocular frame of mind. I thought we'd just made a big mistake.

Meanwhile, on the other end of the phone, when my father told Lima they couldn't have the grain, they wanted it even more. Wow, they thought, this must be really precious. The Americans don't even want to sell it to us.

Lima called back in a couple of weeks or so, and this time I answered the phone. The buyer, Mark Callebert, wanted a truckload of Kamut grain, which was more than we'd sold to anybody at that point. As I often did with our potential partners, I invited Mark to come to my farm to show him what we had. It was late in the year when he arrived in Big Sandy, and the temperature was well below zero. I could tell Mark's coat wasn't quite keeping him warm, but he still wanted to take a look at our crop. I led him out to the bin with our ancient wheat in it, which had a ladder built into the side of it. Mark was game for the climb, so I led the way and opened the door on top of the bin so he could see into it, where our harvested Kamut grain was nearly full to the top. "Very good," Mark said in his thick Flemish accent. "I'll take a third of it."

CHAPTER 7:

A Cowboy in Europe

In 1991, I made my first trip overseas to negotiate an agreement with Lima for introducing Kamut products into Europe. Mark Callebert, the Lima buyer, took me on a big loop. From Lima's headquarters in Belgium, we went to France to talk to cereal companies, then to Italy to talk to pasta manufacturers, then to Switzerland to talk to more cereal companies. I wore my Montana cowboy hat with a head of Kamut grain tucked into the brim, and my hosts introduced me to their local foods, cultures, and natural wonders. It was a blast.

Within a couple of years, we were selling as much ancient wheat in Europe as we were in the United States. I'd signed a five-year exclusive agreement with Lima for the European market. But that no longer seemed like a good idea—for either of us.

One of the most important business lessons I learned in my early years as an entrepreneur had nothing to do with food or agriculture. It was about videotapes. In the late 1970s and early 1980s, home video media started to become enormously popular. From an array of early experiments, two competing formats emerged as the industry's leaders: Video Home System and Betamax.

By 1975, the year before Video Home System launched, Beta-max had the market more or less cornered. Even after its competitor appeared on the scene, there were reasons to think that the Betamax format might remain the popular favorite. It offered higher resolution, a more stable image, and better sound quality than the Video Home System alternative.

Video geeks and business gurus have spilled a lot of ink debating the ins and outs of what happened next. You can really get into the weeds of how these two video formats differ and what the developers did or didn't understand about users' experience. But the part of the story that stood out to me was a key difference in the business strategies pursued by developers of the two formats. Betamax worked exclusively with one manufacturer, Sony. Sony focused heavily on improving picture quality to make home movies look more like movies in theaters. They offered their Betamax tapes in just a single length: one hour. Video Home System made their technology available to any manufacturer who wanted to produce it. This diversity of manufacturers experimented with a number of different improvements to the technology, one of which focused on extending the length of tapes.

As it turned out, length was the feature that mattered most to the everyday people buying videotapes to record their favorite feature films or preserve their children's recitals and basketball games for posterity. Betamax eventually began working with other manufacturers and pro-duced longer tapes, but it was too late. By 1980, Video Home System had captured 60 percent of the North American market. Indeed, "VHS" was becoming so familiar that by the end of the decade, the acronym would become shorthand for "videotape." Meanwhile, Sony's reward for protecting its exclusive arrangement with Betamax through the industry's critical growth years was that they were left holding a very small bag instead of enjoying a piece of a very large pie.[1]

I didn't want to be like Betamax. And I didn't think Lima wanted to be like Sony. So we negotiated an early exit to our exclusive agreement and opened up the European Kamut market to other manufacturers. This was more in line with my philosophy and my experience: while speculative value may increase when you hoard it, real value—to people, communities, and the planet—increases when you *share* it.

Not long after we opened up the European market, Kamut pasta took off in Italy. Italian artisans liked its culinary properties, and naturopathic doctors started recommending it to their patients who were having trouble digesting modern wheat. It spread like wildfire.

Digestive problems with modern wheat weren't unique to Italy; people in the United States were having trouble tolerating it too. But while the physical response to modern wheat may have been similar on either side of the Atlantic, the social response was completely different. In the United States, diet gurus demonized wheat and encouraged people to immediately eliminate it from their meals. Millions of Americans stopped eating bread and pasta, or they ate stuff made with potato flour or some other substitute. Gluten-free products began cropping up in every aisle of the supermarket.

Not in Italy. If you're Italian and you can't eat pasta, it's a problem. Pasta is Italians' heritage, and they don't give it up without a fight. What the Italians understood—especially the naturopathic doctors and the artisanal pasta makers—was that Kamut grain was similar to the wheat that had given birth to their cuisine and their staple foods. *This* was the stuff pasta was supposed to be made out of, not the aggressively bred wheat coming out of the industrial food system that gave people an upset stomach. The problem wasn't wheat. It was what we'd done to it.

Growing grain in the United States and then shipping it to Italy seemed like kind of an ugly American thing to do, and an energy-intensive one at that. Putting so many miles on food was not the business model I'd had in mind. So I looked for someplace closer to the Italian market where I could partner with farmers to grow the ancient wheat. Europe was out—the rainfall was too high for this Mesopotamian crop, and test plots showed susceptibility to disease problems. But right across the Mediterranean was a country where I thought the wheat would feel right at home: Egypt. We had been told that was where it came from, so surely it would thrive there. But that's when I learned a hard lesson about how industrial agriculture had impacted not just American farmers but also farmers in many other parts of the world.

Up until the past century, Egyptian agriculture was fueled by the annual flooding of the Nile River. These seasonal floods brought with them both moisture and nutrient-rich silt, essentially preparing the land for planting. Once the flooding subsided, farmers seeded grain as soon as they could walk in the mud. By the time the fields were running out of moisture, the grain was ripe and ready to harvest. Then the flood season returned and the cycle began again. The ancient Egyptian farmers didn't pay anything for their water, their nutrients, their topsoil. These things just got replenished every year.[2]

But since the building of the Aswan Dams, beginning in 1898 and culminating in 1970 with the completion of the Aswan High Dam, the Nile no longer floods every year. The water has to be purchased. The nutrients have to be purchased. Now Egyptian agriculture is high input—by 1930, the nation was already applying chemical fertilizers at the highest rate per cultivated area in the world[3]—and there is no possibility that its low-output grain could be viable economically. The agriculture has changed so much that the people who preserved and tended this grain for thousands of years can no longer make a living growing it for market. Today, their heirloom grain exists only in small plots for individual consumption, and even those are few and far between in a country that has become reliant on exporting cotton.

This was, of course, one of the chief arguments for building the

Aswan Dams: the new irrigation system allowed colonial administrators to standardize and control Egyptian agriculture in order to facilitate the export of commodity crops—first sugarcane, then cotton. To a Montana wheat farmer, this sounded a lot like the "economic development" strategy that had been forced on my community by the US Department of Agriculture for decades, and, as I would come to understand, this history has been repeated around the world in a global wave of value extraction that continues to this day. Based on the philosophy that specializing in a single cash crop is more economically efficient than growing a diverse mix of products for local use, both physical and economic infrastructure are modified in ways that push farmers to focus exclusively on growing raw materials for export rather than food for their own needs and their region. Impacts on farmers' communities and environments do not figure into the calculus of such a system. Instead, the lens through which value is understood refocuses to a very different spectrum: the gross profits realized throughout the supply chain of whatever monocrop is advised. Frequently, this opening up of commodity markets impoverishes the very areas it promises to develop, as formerly independent communities become dependent on a global market into which they must sell low and from which they must purchase high. Egyptians know all about this: when the fertilizers they came to rely on ran short during World War II (as the same chemicals were diverted to manufacture explosives), they experienced devastating food shortages. While the Egyptian people went hungry, the owners of sugarcane plantations extended their crop's acreage by 30 percent, shipping the country's desperately needed nutrients off to distant lands.[4]

Having learned this sobering lesson about Egyptian agriculture—and the damaging effects of extractive global supply chains—I wondered whether I should continue selling to Italy. It was now my largest market. But given that I was still sourcing grain from North America and shipping it overseas, would I end up doing more harm than good?

To assess the environmental dimension of this question, I commissioned a carbon footprint study. I wanted to know, does grain grown organically in North America and shipped to Italy have a lower carbon footprint than grain grown locally in Italy with chemicals? The answer was yes, a very substantial yes, which surprised me. I couldn't believe the carbon footprint of the agricultural chemicals was enough to cancel out and even exceed the carbon footprint of the long journey over the ocean. But I soon found other studies that came to similar conclusions. The most widely cited was conducted in 2008 by two engineers from Carnegie Mellon University who compared the carbon footprint of "food miles" with the carbon footprint of industrial agricultural practices. According to their findings, food miles—the colloquial term for transportation to final point of sale—account for only about 4 percent of the greenhouse gas emissions associated with the average American diet. Meanwhile, more than 80 percent of the carbon footprint of our diet comes from emissions associated with production.[5] Synthetic fertilizer, as I saw in my own study, is a big part of this story, since its manufacture requires copious amounts of natural gas. So are confinement livestock systems, another major piece of agriculture's climate burden. The bottom line is, if you want to eat sustainably, it makes sense to pay more attention to *how* your food is grown rather than just *where* it's grown.

Being a responsible international business isn't just about greenhouse gas emissions, though. It's also about people. My main concern about growing food in North America and shipping it overseas was that we might undermine the expansion of organic farming in Italy by cutting into Italian growers' markets. The American agricultural-industrial complex has an ugly history of dumping cheap wheat into other countries and putting local farmers out of business.[6] That wasn't the kind of food system I wanted to perpetuate.

Happily, this turned out to be a case of making the organic pie bigger rather than fighting over pieces of it. As Kamut pastas and crackers became more popular in Italy, more and more food artisans wanted to put the ancient wheat in their products. Because of the organic stipulation in our trademark, they couldn't do it without certifying their facilities and ensuring that all the other ingredients in the Kamut products were certified too. All told, 125 Italian companies converted to organic in order to work with Kamut grain. That meant they had to find someone who could supply them with organic oil, yeast, or whatever other ingredients they needed for their creations. Some even started making additional organic items, beyond their Kamut products, to make the most of the investment they'd made to certify their facilities. As a result, the market for Italian organic farmers has actually expanded since we started exporting our ancient wheat over there.

As I was working through these dilemmas with the Kamut supply chain, one thing was still bugging me. Being a scientist, I wanted to verify the legends about "King Tut's wheat." Could the seeds of this grain really have come from King Tut's tomb, as the guy had said at the Fort Benton County Fair?

By this time, I knew how the grain had gotten to Montana. In 1949, an Air Force transport pilot from a farm near Fort Benton had gotten thirty-six seeds from a fellow serviceman at a base in Portugal. The seeds came with an intriguing legend: the serviceman claimed to have gotten them from an excavated tomb while on a furlough in Egypt. The Montana airman mailed the seeds to his father, who planted them on the family farm and began spreading their progeny around the community. The local newspaper ran a story about this "King Tut wheat" in 1964, faithfully reproducing the legend passed down from the airman to his father to the mailman who circulated the seeds to their neighbors.[7] Like everyone else in Central Montana, the man who showed me the grain at the county fair had taken this secondhand story at face value. And, at first, so had I.

But I had my doubts. I had been hearing from researchers that it was impossible for four-thousand-year-old grain to germinate. A paleobotanist from the East Coast sent me some grain that she had taken out of a tomb in Egypt, as the serviceman claimed to have done with the seed stock of our ancient wheat. I opened the envelope and pulled out a shriveled gray kernel, which disintegrated to dust when I squeezed it between my fingers. The rest of the seeds were in much the same condition: completely dried out and easily reduced to a fine powder. Okay, I thought, maybe the serviceman didn't get the grain *directly* from a tomb. But maybe it was handed down from the time of the pharaohs and some local farmer in Egypt sold it at the market with a story.

The first chance I had to travel to Egypt, in 1997, I went to the museum in Cairo and found an exhibit on the age of the pharaohs. The exhibit had wheat in it, which was encouraging. But the grain in the exhibit looked to me like einkorn, an even older ancient wheat that has a very distinctive shape and striations along the kernel. It certainly wasn't the variety I was growing.

That trip to Egypt left me even more confused. Where *did* this wheat come from? And just what was it? A lab in North Dakota told me it was *Triticum polonicum*, Polish wheat. A lab in Oregon told me it was *Triticum turanicum*, khorasan wheat. The N. I. Vavilov Institute of Plant Genetic Resources in St. Petersburg, Russia, told me it might be a type of durum—the kind of wheat used for making pasta rather than bread. But the Russians also told me something else: I wasn't asking quite the right question. The sample I'd sent them was not a pure variety, they told me, but a "landrace."

Before plant breeding became a specialized occupation, farmers selected their own seeds in the field, replanting the ones from the crops that weathered the storms or bore the tastiest fruit or grew the tallest—typically some combination of all the traits they wanted. But instead of narrowing this genetic pool to the single best specimen—as is often done now—our forefarmers built some insurance into this system of genetic selection. Instead of planting identical monocultures, they gathered closely related lines and planted them together in the field. If disaster struck, in the form of disease or insects or unusual weather, some of the plants would be more resistant than others, so the farmers wouldn't lose everything. Instead, the surviving plants would grow bigger and fill in the spaces left by the failed ones, ensuring adequate food at harvest. These mixed plantings sometimes cross-pollinated and were in a constant state of gradual genetic evolution. Thus, our forefarmers' crops didn't consist of single plant varieties as we understand the term today. They were genetically heterogenous strains: landraces.

This clever genetic strategy of landraces was based on a fundamental principle of ecology: mixture. Look at a pasture, look at a forest. Nature never farms in monocultures. If there's one word that should be on the mind of every farmer, it should be "diversity." And I think it extends beyond the farm field too, whether you're talking about a business or a club or any sort of organization. The more diverse it is, the more resilient it is, because you've got all these different talents, you've got all these different viewpoints. It's more complex. It may not be as easy to manage. But when a problem comes down the pike, you're more likely to have someone in the mix who has a solution to it. Or, better yet, someone who's anticipated the problem and headed it off at the pass.

I thought it was good news that the ancient wheat I was growing was a genetically diverse landrace, and it made sense to me because of its resistance to drought and sawflies. But I still felt like part of the story was missing. Where did it come from?

Then, in 2007, I traveled to Turkey to experiment with growing the grain over there. (I was still looking for options closer to Italy.) That didn't really work, but at the first company we visited, the owner nodded in recognition when I showed him the seeds. "Ah, yes," he said. "We know this grain. We call it Camel Tooth." He proceeded to explain the reasoning behind the name: the grain was big on one end and small on the other, with a hump shape. Hmm, I thought. I guess it sort of looks like a tooth.

"Or the other name," the owner of the Turkish company continued, before I could fully visualize a camel's tooth, "is the Prophet's Wheat."

"The Prophet's Wheat," I asked. "Did it have something to do with Muhammad?"

"Oh, no, no, no," he said, shaking his finger. "Not that prophet. You know, the one with the boat."

The one with the boat? I turned that over in my head. "Do you mean Noah?"

"Yes," the man replied. "This is the grain that Noah brought with him on the Ark."

I can't verify whether there were any Kamut grains on Noah's Ark. But after my trip to Turkey, I did finally get a definitive lab identification, which determined that it is khorasan wheat, that it is a landrace, and that it originated in Mesopotamia. I've since found many other references to Camel Tooth wheat across the region, from Turkey to Palestine, all of which look like the wheat I grow.

Now I knew the truth: our grain was native to Mesopotamia, not to Egypt. It wouldn't have made it into Africa during the time of the pharaohs, so it couldn't have been in King Tut's tomb—or any tomb. This grain that became a staple of Egyptian agriculture had come to the region later, probably a couple thousand years later. With traders.

At the Fort Benton County Fair, a man had captured my imagination with an exotic story about a grain from ancient Egypt, a grain so quintessentially Egyptian that it had been found in King Tut's tomb. The story, I had discovered, was false. Just a tale told at a carnival, no doubt embellished in the retelling. But, more importantly, the larger story was false. To imagine the genetic basis of agriculture as a static archive of pure varieties, frozen in time and place, was to misunderstand the dynamic relationship between seeds and their farmers, the constant interplay of nature and culture. It was to forget that trade has been part of this interplay all along, from the spices carried along the Silk Road to the Peruvian potatoes that became the national pride of Ireland. We've been exchanging seeds all along.

Now, of course, that global exchange has been put in service of the same commodity mentality that I encountered as it began devastating my wheat-farming community in Montana. In response, a number of people seeking to repair the integrity of the food system have called for an end to its globalization. Declaring themselves locavores, many of these people have pledged to eat only food grown within a hundred-mile radius of their homes.

There's a real need to revitalize local and regional food systems in many parts of the world, and I've made this a major part of my focus in the past couple decades of my career. But drawing a hundred-mile radius around our community? That seems out of step with humanity's history of global exchange and the many valuable and delicious creations that have come of it. I don't think we should abolish this exchange. But I think we should become far more attentive to its terms, to ensure that balance and diversity are maintained and value is provided for everyone along the way.

By 2017, our Kamut khorasan was being grown by almost two hundred family farms on a total of approximately one hundred thousand acres of certified organic cropland, mostly in Montana and Saskatchewan. Seventy-five percent of that grain was bound for Italy. Shipping food across oceans wasn't our original intent, but since we're faced with an industrial food system that's eviscerated regional infrastructure and culinary traditions, we have to start rebuilding these foundations piece by piece, recognizing that the whole puzzle won't come together all at once. The corporate commodity system has spent decades sidelining human health, rural livelihoods, and the viability of the planet in the name of cheap food and obscene profits. We won't turn it around in one year or with one business. But we might turn it around with a sustained global effort to model the future we want while working to change the laws and incentives that favor the status quo. If you're truly committed to the values of sustainable business, you can't just be an entrepreneur. You also have to be an active citizen.

CHAPTER 8:

Creating a New Standard

When you're the chapter president of the leading organic certifier in your region and the entire statewide membership is sitting around your kitchen table, you don't think of organics as an industry. And in the mid-1980s, it really wasn't. Whole Foods Market was still just a local grocery store in Austin, Texas, with two new satellite locations in Dallas and Houston. Earthbound Farms was a two-and-a-half-acre backyard raspberry farm.

But in February 1989, CBS's *60 Minutes* broadcast a program about the dangers of Alar, a chemical commonly sprayed on apples to regulate growth and enhance color. The Natural Resources Defense Council had recently issued a report finding that the cumulative effect of repeated exposure to Alar could cause cancer. Americans were stunned. And terrified.

The only way to be sure an apple wasn't sprayed with Alar was to buy organic. So people did. In droves. Other exposés about the chemicals in industrial food followed. When Americans found out that conventional dairies were using recombinant bovine growth hormone, organic milk sales soared. Organics spread from co-ops to supermarkets, from hippies to yuppies. Beginning in the 1990s, total organic sales grew by double digits each year: 20 percent, 30 percent. And they never stopped.

For those of us in the organic farming community, this was exciting. And also perilous. As organics began to look like big business, new players entered the industry, some of whom were in it just to make a quick buck. In the frenzied environment that was early 1990s organics, I was very worried that our nascent industry might go the way of our predecessor, natural foods.

"Natural food" used to mean something. Back in the early days of the food show I went to every year in Anaheim—Natural Products Expo West—it was kind of like "organic." Whole foods. Minimally processed. Grown without chemicals or hormones. Why bother with a legal definition for something so self-evident? But by the early 1990s, as demand rose, people were trying to pawn off all sorts of ridiculous things as "all natural." It was a joke. I didn't want to see "organic" get co-opted and watered down like that, and with Johnny-come-lately organic manufacturers angling to lower their cost of production, the threat seemed imminent.

In fairness, the organic world of the late 1980s wasn't completely the Wild West. Not like it was in 1984, when I started going around asking Montana wheat farmers to "self-certify" by signing affidavits that said they were following the California organic standard. By the late 1980s, there were many reputable certifiers in operation all over the country, conducting thorough organic inspections. The problem was, every single one had a different standard—and some states had no standard. There was constant bickering about whose standard was more stringent, and I could imagine that if a less reputable certifier were to enter the game and try to undercut everybody else, the whole organic industry could collapse under the weight of infighting. In order to protect the value we'd worked so hard to create and to establish a fair set of rules for everybody, I came to believe, we needed to move into the arena of public policy.

So in the late 1980s, I joined a group of fellow organic farmers and advocates in petitioning Congress to include a formal definition of "organic" in the 1990 Farm Bill. To the surprise of many, Congress listened, and the Organic Foods Production Act of 1990 was included in the massive package of agricultural legislation and signed into law. The law, however, was just a framework. The details of the new federal organic standard would need to be fleshed out by the agency in charge of enforcing the law, the US Department of Agriculture.

This was clearly a case where the devil was in the details, so in 1990, I accepted my peers' nomination and was appointed by the secretary of agriculture to serve on the USDA's first ever National Organic Standards Board. It was our job to advise the agency on a single set of standards for organics, which would become the law of the land.

My fellow board members and I spent two years traveling around the country, gathering as much information and input as we could from farmers, manufacturers, and eaters of organic food. We wrestled with tough questions about what it truly meant to be organic. Was it okay to bring in fertilizer from off the farm, as long as it hadn't been manufactured in a chemical process? What if that naturally occurring fertilizer had to be mined and shipped across the ocean? Even tougher questions arose when we had to define what "organic" meant for a processed product, like pasta sauce or pretzels. Would we allow organic food manufacturers to use chemical soap to clean the equipment in their factory? What about the lye needed to create the crusty sheen on a pretzel?

After months of deliberation, we wrote up our recommendations and sent them off to the USDA. The agency took a year to study them. We thought, Boy, they are taking this seriously. As the date approached for the agency to announce its rule, I made plans to fly to Washington, DC, for the occasion. My term on the board had ended at that point, but I figured this was an important milestone in the organic movement. I didn't want to miss the celebration.

And yet, when our little assembly of organic advocates got our hands on a preliminary draft of the proposed rule, the jovial mood quickly vanished. Under its proposed definition of "organic," the USDA was going to allow irradiation, GMOs—even sewage sludge.[1]

My fellow board members and I were irate. We'd spent the better part of a decade trying to put organics on firmer footing—and now it appeared that this federal rule was going to erode the movement entirely. The USDA's proposed standard was hardly a standard at all. It watered down the whole idea of organic to the point that the term was almost meaningless.

But what could we do? Clearly, the USDA wasn't listening to us. It didn't appear that our congresspeople were going to go to bat for us, either. We had exhausted all our channels of influence.

Except one. Thanks to the Administrative Procedure Act of 1946, federal agencies have to provide a public comment period before finalizing a proposed rule. That was our window of opportunity: ninety days. And in a fortunate twist of fate, this would be one of the first such comment periods that would allow input through a newly available channel: the internet.[2]

The chair of the National Organic Standards Board at that time, Michael Sligh, gathered a small group to analyze the federal rule and identify all the points on which it diverged from our recommendations. The group titled its analysis "The Sixty-Six Points of Darkness"—a play on the George H. W. Bush administration's Thousand Points of Light initiative. These sixty-six points of darkness—our list of objections to the USDA rule—were widely circulated through email lists and postcard campaigns, reaching farmer organizations, consumer groups, certifying bodies, and a host of organic food retailers and processors. These groups circulated the sixty-six points to their members, publicizing the opportunity for public comment. By the time the comment period closed, the USDA had received more than 275,000 comments—more than they'd received for any other rule in the agency's history. The overwhelming majority came from eaters of organic food, and they were not favorable.[3] "Allow us the choice of true organic foods," one commenter wrote, in all capital letters. "Don't give us the same old crap and call it organic."[4]

Near the end of the comment period, Michael Sligh went down to the USDA sub-basement, where the public feedback was being collected and tallied. He found a beleaguered group of young staffers stacking page after page of comments, visibly exhausted from the work. "Can you make them stop?" one of the staffers pleaded, when he told them who he was. "Of course I can't stop it," Michael replied. "I have no control over this thing. This thing has a life of its own. There's nobody in charge! You have now, you know, unleashed this thing. The only way you're going to deal with it is you're going to have to withdraw the rule and get it right."[5]

To its credit, the USDA listened. When the National Organic Program was finally rolled out in 2000, irradiation, GMOs, and sewage sludge were all prohibited. The outcome of the National Organic Program rule was a huge win for democracy, and I think the final version demonstrates that our government can be made to live up to Abe Lincoln's admonition that it be of the people, by the people, and for the people. But the process taught me some hard lessons.

During the years I served on the National Organic Standards Board, I saw firsthand how much influence the agricultural-industrial complex has on our government. Industry almost got irradiated GMOs grown with sewage sludge into the organic program, for crying out loud. And the battle is never over—Big Food is always lobbying for some chemical or another to be placed on the list of organically approved inputs. Similar stories can be told about the ongoing battles over the food pyramid and federal dietary recommendations[6] or about agricultural chemicals that have been banned in Europe but are still legal here.[7] The food and agricultural industry has enormous power to shape decisions that are supposed to be made in the public interest.

Monopolies are nothing new under the sun. Big Oil. Big Railroads. Big Meatpackers. People have been fighting for generations to "break up the trusts," as my grandfather's contemporaries would have said. Going way back to our earliest days as a nation, Americans have believed that it's not fair for one person or organization to have so much power that they diminish possibilities for others to prosper and flourish. And going way back, it's been a struggle to defend that principle.

But now we have multinational corporations that are bigger than some governments. And their goal is to make even more money and increase their power and control. If you look at recent consolidation in the food industry, even the organic food industry, it's abundantly clear that big players are pushing the little players out of the market—or buying them up. As a result, just ten companies control a significant portion of the world food supply.[8]

Professor Phil Howard at Michigan State University makes diagrams of this consolidation—with big colorful circles representing the large corporations buying everybody out and little drab ovals representing the companies getting acquired.[9] Arrows connect all the little drab ovals to the big colorful circles that have swallowed them up. It's a bit of an ironic picture, since it's the companies represented by the big bright circles that are making our landscapes, our crops, and our diets so much *less* colorful. But those ballooning red and yellow orbs certainly grab your attention.

On the diagram for the seed industry, you can see that just six colorful circles—Monsanto, Syngenta, DuPont, Bayer, BASF, and Dow—have acquired 317 little drab ovals. In only seventeen years. Since Professor Howard created this graphic, Dow and DuPont have merged, Bayer has acquired Monsanto, and ChemChina has acquired Syngenta.[10] If all those mergers hold up in court, these three mega-corporations will control 59 percent of the global seed market and 64 percent of pesticides.[11]

A similar fate has befallen food retail (four chains control 50 percent of US sales),[12] beef (four corporations control 80 percent of US cattle),[13] poultry (five firms sell 70 percent of chicken consumed in the United States),[14] dairy (the four largest co-ops plus Dean Foods capture 80 percent of US fluid milk sales),[15] and pork (four corporations control 66 percent of US hogs).[16] Global commodities—wheat, corn, soy, rice, palm oil, sugar—are controlled by just four firms that account for 70 percent of the market: Archer Daniels Midland, Bunge, Cargill, and the Louis Dreyfus Company, or simply "ABCD."[17] But to me, the most sobering case of consolidation is the one threatening the integrity of the organic industry. On Phil Howard's diagram of organics, many of the big colorful circles have merged, leaving just thirty independent clusters in place of what were once the top one hundred organic food processors. One of those colorful circles, the Hain Celestial Group, has swallowed up a whopping twenty-seven little drab ovals in just twenty years. Among the organic companies that have recently been acquired is Dave's Killer Bread, an organic bakery that bought wheat from many of my fellow farmers in Montana. In 2015, it was purchased by Flowers Foods, the maker of Wonder Bread.[18]

Big Food's consolidation is an obvious problem for eaters and small businesses, but it's also been devastating for farmers, who've steadily sacrificed more and more of their earnings to marketers and input suppliers. In 1910, farmers accounted for 41 percent of the economic activity within the agricultural sector. By 1990, that figure was down to 9 percent. Meanwhile, the share of that economic activity captured by input suppliers shot up from 15 percent to 24 percent; marketers captured a whopping 67 percent, up from 44 percent at the turn of the twentieth century. One result of this flip-flop in value is that agricultural input suppliers and food marketers have become some of the largest corporations in the world. And the other result is that farmers earn less in real income than they did in 1910.[19]

The problem isn't just scale. It's not that big companies are inherently bad and little companies are inherently good. The important thing is the nature of the company's business model. Is the company extracting value or adding it? Recently, a handful of mainstream food corporations have been showing up at organic meetings and asking us how they can be part of the solution. This is what I tell them: Look at your business model. Are you structured to extract value out of communities and into commodities? Because to my thinking, that's not organic. Organic— real organic—requires a whole systems approach, with value regenerated at every stage in the process. This is how we farm, and this is also how we do business.

In the past, Big Organic has mostly gone the extractive commodity route. But I'm encouraged to see some companies working to shift their business models to serve all their stakeholders, not just shareholders. From what I've seen so far, these companies don't build their businesses on the backs of somebody else. Quite the opposite, in fact: they want to share their success. This is what we've tried to do with the Kamut project.

If you were to look at the total value of the Kamut products produced in a year—the amount of money that people ultimately pay when they buy the ancient wheat in a box of pasta or a loaf of bread—it would be a multimillion-dollar operation. But very little of that passes through my hands. The farmers own the grain. They sell it to a cleaning plant— either Montana Flour and Grains in Fort Benton or Prairie Heritage Seeds Organics in Radville, Saskatchewan. The cleaning plant sells it to a mill, which sells it to someone who makes pasta or bread or crackers out of it. Then they sell it to a retailer or a restaurateur. All the while it's gaining value and paying bills for people. To me, that is a good business. That is a successful business.

When my son was in high school in Big Sandy, he loved basketball. He wasn't a star athlete, but he was a solid member of the group. Hard worker. Team player. He had a genuine enjoyment of the game that was infectious, so he got everybody fired up.

But the coach only cared about his top five players. He focused on his top five players because that's who he thought would win him state championships. My son wasn't in the top five, so he hardly ever got to play. In high school? Come on. It should be for the fun of the game, getting all the kids involved, teaching life skills, communication, working together—all those wonderful things about team sports.

If you look in the award case at Big Sandy High School, it's loaded with basketball trophies. But they came at a pretty high cost to all those kids who were sidelined. As I see it, that's where we are in the food industry. You've got a few companies hell-bent on being champions of everything, at any cost.

What that means for the rest of us is that we can't just assume our government is going to maintain a level playing field when it comes to food, agriculture, and the myriad ways in which our food system impacts our lives. We can't assume that our public officials are going to be perfect referees and ensure everyone plays fair. We have to constantly hold them accountable and call foul if they don't.

One thing we really have to watch out for is loopholes in our laws— which often result when lawyers write convoluted legislation that can be interpreted only by a large corporation with a bevy of lawyers on staff. In our attempt to codify organic practices for the purposes of the National Organic Program, we in the organic community sometimes fell prey to these kinds of legal rat's nests, which can have the unintended effect of being overly burdensome for small farmers who are most closely following the spirit of the law but least equipped to document that they are following it in letter. This was a major concern of our board when it came to one of the thorniest aspects of the organic rule: livestock confinement. The question at hand sounded simple, but it quickly got complex: is it organic to raise animals indoors?

At one of the National Organic Program meetings I attended, somebody made the point that if we didn't allow confinement of cattle in the winter, when the pastures are all muddy, it could ruin the land and sicken the cattle. That made sense to me—give the animals shelter in extreme weather. People need shelter in extreme weather.

But when you extend that to chickens, a chicken's entire life span can occur in the winter. If a chicken is raised in confinement during the winter, it's organic, but if it's raised in confinement during the summer, it's not organic? That never made much sense to me.

Meanwhile, we also got a big debate going about another livestock rule, on antibiotics. On conventional factory farms, antibiotics are used as a matter of course to prevent animals from getting sick under such unhealthy conditions. This routine use of antibiotics has led to a rise in antibiotic-resistant bacteria, which are a threat not only to livestock but also to humans. The organic community has been united against this practice, and we've all decided that routine use of antibiotics is not something that should be allowed under our standard. But, some asked, what about when an individual animal gets sick? Could we somehow write the regulation to distinguish routine antibiotic use from therapeutic antibiotic use?

This is the sort of thing that drives me crazy. Here we were in one room discussing how to regulate antibiotic use. Then, in another room, a different group of us was debating how many square feet a chicken needs to be happy.

My argument was, if you eliminate the possibility of using antibiotics, farmers are going to do everything they can to be sure that their animals are not getting sick. Animals, just like people, become susceptible to disease when they are stressed. And confinement causes stress.

Let the chicken tell you how many square feet it needs. Because if it doesn't have enough, it's going to get stressed, and it's going to get sick. As long as we don't cover up the problem with antibiotics, farmers will solve it.

I never got much traction with that proposal. But after seven years of deliberation, the organic community put together a thoughtfully worded animal welfare rule to ensure that there were no loopholes that would allow livestock raised in confinement to be sold as organic. With broad support, it was finalized by the USDA in 2016. Many people thought that might be the end of it. And yet, a year later, a new administration proposed a withdrawal of the rule. Despite receiving over 70,000 public comments, overwhelmingly in support of the animal welfare standards, this new USDA struck them from the books. A handful of corporate organic egg producers and confinement dairies are delighted. But a coalition of organic and animal welfare groups are suing.[20] We aren't just going to sit back and let the USDA water down the standards we've worked so hard to build.

I still think the National Organic Program was a good idea. Although it wasn't perfectly executed, I think it continues to serve its purpose in protecting the integrity of the organic standard. When you see the USDA Organic Seal, you can be confident that no synthetic pesticides or fertilizers were used to produce your food. That alone won't fix the food system, but it's a very meaningful contribution to human health and the health of the planet.

These days, a number of folks are talking about "regenerative agriculture" and proposing this concept as a new benchmark of sustainability. I'm glad this idea is being widely circulated, as I think it's a good reminder of the principle at the heart of organic. We can't just settle for substituting one set of inputs with a less toxic set of inputs. We actually have to design self-regenerating farm systems—which also regenerate the planet and rural communities. But if organic needs regenerative, the reverse is also true. No farming system should call itself regenerative if it relies on polluting chemicals. So rather than create a new standard or a new label, I think the regenerative agriculture movement should build on the organic standard. It's earned our customers' trust for a reason.

But like all public programs, the National Organic Program needs active public support—and scrutiny. We, the public, have to ensure that the program is funded to do its job, and we also have to hold it accountable. We can't give up if we don't get traction right away. We have to keep showing up at meetings and commenting on proposed rules, like all those people did in 1998 when the USDA tried to sneak in irradiation and GMOs and sewage sludge. We have to call foul. Or fowl, in the case of confined chickens. Otherwise, Big Food will bend the whole thing to boost its profit margins and "organic" won't mean anything anymore.

Although I've spent my entire career in business and am often frustrated by bureaucratic government programs, I have come to accept the fact that there are some things we can't leave to the private sector alone. Current federal policy disadvantages the value-added economy in important ways—letting Big Food off the hook for the costs it imposes on the rest of us. If we don't work to change it, the deck will always be stacked against us.

CHAPTER 9:

The Value of Limits

In 1999, I told my wife I was ready to slow down. I was fifty years old. I'd been in business for twenty years. After a long, slow climb to pay off the debt from my initial investment, my flour mill was making some real money. My goal had been to provide a new market for our farm and other organic farmers in the state, to prove that you could make a living without either the chemical treadmill or the commodity system. I felt like I'd accomplished that.

So that year, I sold Montana Flour and Grains to my chief financial officer, André Giles. I still wanted to do more work with ancient wheat—particularly research on the nutrition aspects—so I held onto that part of the business under the name Kamut International.

I was letting go of a profitable operation just as it started to grow, but I'd never intended Montana Flour and Grains to be a cash cow. I had wanted it to be a solid community business, and it was. It had created ten good jobs in the little town of Fort Benton and would now be locally owned by André, a Little League coach whose wife, Karyn, had poured her heart and soul into local efforts to recycle, raise awareness about breast cancer, care for stray animals, and organize community concerts.

Part of me wanted that to be enough—why not call it two decades of a job well done and semi-retire to my farm? I told all my friends and family that I was selling Montana Flour and Grains so I could simplify my life. But there was still so much work to do. Particularly right here in Big Sandy.

Like many farming communities in the United States, Big Sandy suffers from an ironic dearth of healthy, fresh food. Since nearly all our farmland grows commodity grain that gets shipped *out*, most of the food we eat has to get shipped *in*. Shipping food in is expensive, in both economic and environmental terms, but we have come to rely on these imports of standard American groceries—wintertime tomatoes, bananas, avocados—most of which are sourced from areas with longer growing seasons and more water, from either the sky or irrigation. It's not a very sustainable system, and it leaves much of our region hungry. We're not alone: a recent analysis of the 314 most food-insecure counties in the United States found that over three-quarters of them are rural. Child hunger in America is even more concentrated in the countryside. When the same researchers looked specifically at the counties with the highest levels of food insecurity among children, they found that 86 percent of these are classified as rural.[1]

I wanted Big Sandy to be able to grow the fruits and vegetables that our kids were lacking. But, like most things in my career, my "retirement" project didn't start with a grand plan. Just like my foray into organic grain, it began with a simple experiment.

I was looking for something to do with the saline seep on my farm. These seeps are pockets of salty groundwater, which eventually destroy your ability to grow crops. As saline water builds up over time, the water comes to the surface and then evaporates, leaving behind white salt crystals. It's a problem that's skyrocketed in recent years as irrigation and bare fallowed land have combined to create more of these salty pools.

During the 1970s, Montanans reported a nearly fourfold increase in cropland destroyed by seeps, from 51,000 acres to 200,000 acres.[2]

Over the years, I had learned that planting alfalfa surrounding the saline areas can help dry up the seeps, drawing water away before the salty solution breaks above the surface of the ground. This stops salt from accumulating on the land, giving rain a chance to wash the already accumulated salts back through the soil. Eventually, the salinity in the seep area gets back to normal, so you can grow plants there again. But it's a long process, five to ten years. (This is yet another reason why it's a good idea to plant cover crops—they can catch excess moisture and utilize it, so you never get to the seep stage of things.) So I thought, Why don't we try growing something there that *needs* more water? Like vegetables.

In the spring of 2007, I planted vegetables straight across the seep to find out where they'd be most successful. I saw it as a Goldilocks problem. In the center, it would be too salty. On the far edge, it would be too dry. But somewhere in between might be just right. I planted vegetables that I thought might grow successfully without irrigation: potatoes, onions, squash. As I was taught in college, every good experiment needs a control. So I also planted a bunch of these same vegetables a quarter mile away from the seep, out in the middle of a dry field.

My Goldilocks hypothesis was sort of right. The plants in the center of the seep looked pretty sorry, and so did the ones on the edge. There was a very narrow band somewhere in between where they looked a little better.

But the real story of the experiment was the control. The vegetables that I'd planted out in the middle of my dry field did much better than any of the ones in the trial plots. They looked almost as good as the plants in my garden.

I was amazed. To think you could grow vegetables without irrigation on thirteen inches of annual precipitation! I shouldn't have been so shocked, though, because the homesteaders grew vegetables without irrigation. My grandparents had a little garden out back, where my grain bins are now, which certainly would not have been irrigated. The experiment station nearby in Havre had maintained a trial plot of dryland potatoes up through the time I came back to the farm, which I recalled seeing on a field visit there. Once I began jogging my memory and studying dryland vegetables, I learned that many other people have been doing this successfully for centuries. In areas with astonishingly little water.

In a 1910 book on the potential of dry farming, agricultural scientist John Widtsoe marveled at the fact that the ancient city of Tunis received just nine inches of rainfall per year and left no evidence of irrigation. Yet, Widtsoe noted, archaeologists had found ruins of an ancient Tunisian amphitheater large enough to accommodate 60,000 people.[3] Without rain or irrigation, what were all those people eating?

Hard as it is to believe from the vantage point of today's heavily irrigated American agriculture, the Tunisian experience was not an anomaly. In fact, many Mediterranean societies still dry-farm numerous crops: olives, grapes, figs, apricots, walnuts, almonds.[4] In some parts of Europe, it's illegal to irrigate wine grapes in the middle of the growing season, on the grounds that too much water would dilute the quality of the grapes. In addition to fruit trees and grains, California farmers also dry-farm potatoes, cantaloupes, watermelons, and tomatoes.[5] The tomatoes, in particular, have been quite successful. Beginning with the pioneering Molino Creek Farming Collective, near Santa Cruz, farmers on California's Central Coast have developed a specialty market for dry-farmed tomatoes, which chefs and market-goers prize for their intense flavor.

I've continued my own experiments with non-irrigated vegetables. I started with twenty-four varieties of squash and found four that are adapted for life on the prairie. I tried forty varieties of potatoes and ended up with five that really do well here. What amazed me about these crops was that if I gave them three times as much space as recommended for raising them in an irrigated garden, they produced equivalent yields on a plant-per-plant basis. All they needed was a little more room to go out and find the water they needed underground—and I had to keep an eye out for weeds, so that uninvited plants didn't steal any of the subsurface moisture. My farm was becoming my garden.

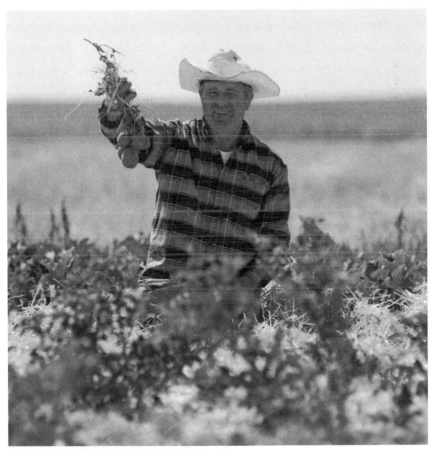

HARVESTING DRYLAND POTATOES FROM MY EXPERIMENTAL TEST PLOT.
(Photo by Sean Knighton)

Some of my potato varieties are better mashers, while some are better bakers. Some of them are "short keepers"—they break dormancy early in the season and grow quickly, so they are the first ones on our plates. Some are "long keepers"—they need warmer temperatures to break dormancy, which means they mature more slowly but keep longer once they are harvested. All this diversity means I can harvest a perfectly adequate complement of diverse produce on our north central Montana dryland throughout the growing season. Then, in winter, we have our storage vegetables, fresh from the root cellar.

A root cellar is very low-cost storage. I have one little fan in mine to circulate the air, and it doesn't cost even a penny a day. This simple structure keeps our potatoes fresh from October to early July, when the first potatoes of our next year's crop are ready. Other root vegetables, like carrots and beets, will keep in the root cellar until April, and we store winter squash in garage cupboards until midsummer, when our summer squash is ready to be picked. Onions can be stored fresh until about January. Then we move the remainder to our freezer to tide us over to the next harvest. In this way, we can eat quality produce all year round without ever having to buy something that's shipped in—or pay for irrigation. The one thing we can't farm on dryland is off-season vegetables. But I don't need to eat watermelon twelve months a year.

I think dryland vegetables are very important for the future of agriculture because of our looming water crisis. Already, 1.2 billion people—almost 20 percent of the global population—live in areas of physical water scarcity, meaning that current withdrawals use over 75 percent of river flows. Another 500 million people live in areas approaching this condition, and yet another 1.6 billion live in areas of economic water scarcity, due to infrastructure or inequitable distribution. That's half the world worried about where their water is going to come from.[6]

With so much pressure on surface water, people are increasingly looking underground. Groundwater depletion rates doubled between 1960 and 2000, with 67 percent of that water going to agriculture.[7] Rising global temperatures will exacerbate these problems, intensifying the water cycle. As the Intergovernmental Panel on Climate Change put it, "Water and its availability and quality will be the main pressures on, and issues for, societies and the environment under climate change."[8]

Cities and households are already being asked to conserve water in many parts of the United States and around the world, but increasingly, the global community is looking to farmers to achieve greater water conservation. With agriculture accounting for over 70 percent of global freshwater use,[9] we can't solve the water problem without rethinking irrigation. Within a few decades, our farming systems may need to adapt to far less supplemental water than we currently use.

But even in the near term, I think a dryland vegetable operation could be a great business for farm families in places like Big Sandy. Imagine if every town in the upper Great Plains had a few surrounding farms that supplied the population with most of their basic vegetables. Land that doesn't have access to irrigation is cheaper. You don't have the added expense of water or the energy required to pump it. And you don't have all the costs associated with putting miles on food—trucking and refrigerated storage and all of that.

For someone in the situation I was in forty years ago—for a young parent who wants to come back to the family farm—this could be the answer. You don't have to go into enormous debt. You don't have to expand the farm and buy out your neighbors. You can add a high-value enterprise and support two families on the same piece of land. I've been trialing this approach on my own farm, where a young farmer now earns part of his living running our dryland vegetable operation.

The other thing some of my friends noticed about my dryland vegetables was their intense flavor. It was as if I'd taken orange juice concentrate and added only half the recommended water. Then I realized this might not be far from the truth: these vegetables, quite literally, had not been watered down. If the flavors were so concentrated, I wondered, what might this mean for the nutrient content? Researchers in my own field of plant biochemistry had been looking at this question for decades, finding that plants experience something called the "dilution effect."[10]

"The more water available to a plant, the faster it will grow, the bigger the fruit will become, the higher the moisture content in the harvest," explains Dr. Charles Benbrook, an agricultural economist at Johns Hopkins University. "When there is plenty of available nitrogen too, the carbohydrate levels in the plant—basically, sugar water—will go through the roof. All of the above dilute the presence of other nutrients."[11]

Benbrook further explains that plants with excess supplies of water and nutrients have to do something with these resources, and converting them into carbohydrates is the easiest option, since this poses the least energetic cost to the plant. But it's not necessarily the best option for us.

The wine industry, Benbrook notes, has already discovered that reducing or eliminating irrigation produces higher-quality wines with higher levels of phenols and antioxidants—compounds that plants release in response to stress that have been linked to cancer prevention and other health benefits. Benbrook believes that agricultural science should be much more focused on how to boost levels of such health-promoting compounds in our food plants.[12] But unfortunately, we've mostly been going in the opposite direction.

In 2004, a biochemist from the University of Texas at Austin, Dr. Don Davis, published an analysis of changes in nutrient density for forty-three crops. Between 1950 and 1999, Davis found, US Department of Agriculture data showed significant declines in the median concentrations of six nutrients: protein, calcium, phosphorus, iron, riboflavin, and vitamin C.[13] So what changed in half a century?

It's hard to tease out the influence of several different factors on these declines in nutrient density, Benbrook explains, but it comes down to three major culprits. Irrigation, as I'd suspected after eating my own dryland vegetables. Nitrogen fertilizer, which plays an even larger role in the environmental dilution effect, boosting plants' carbohydrate ratios even higher. And plant breeding, which has selected for varieties that produce higher yields rather than higher nutrient content.[14] Here was another clue about my friend Laura's seemingly miraculous experience eating Kamut pasta. This was an ancient crop grown on dryland without synthetic nitrogen fertilizer.

I had started my dryland vegetable experiment as a salvage operation for my saline seeps. But I ended up learning two major lessons from my plants: There are serious benefits to living within your limits. And there is so much we can do with what we already have.

In my lifetime, the objective of agricultural research and industry has mostly been to overcome nature's limits: tame, conquer, subdue. But as I saw with my dryland vegetables, the real opportunity is in working *within* limits: non-irrigated produce holds the potential to eliminate our dependence on both imported food and dwindling water resources. Even the plants themselves develop a more balanced nutrient profile when they live within their limits, which means better nutrition for all of us who eat them. Unfortunately, it's hard to see these "less is more" opportunities, because the commodity food system is totally geared toward gross rather than net. American agriculture has been so busy patting itself on the back for high production that we have ignored its high cost, which is often subsidized in some fashion. The result is that we've greatly neglected opportunities for net gain: opportunities that come from working within limits, minimizing input costs, and learning when enough is enough. When we shift our perspective from gross to net, we can start finding truly elegant solutions for meeting our needs without undermining our future.

By now I had a pretty good idea of how to sustainably supply grain to my community in Big Sandy, and I'd taken a key step toward community food security with my dryland vegetables, which are now served at the Big Sandy Senior Center and sold by local grocery stores and restaurants. Many of my Montana neighbors had become nationwide leaders in the grass-finished beef movement, and a company not far away was processing and marketing organic lentils, so we were well on our way to sustainable sources of protein. But the missing link, the item that everybody, including me, still imported from thousands of miles away, was fruit. Except for a few berries and crab apples, this key food group was notably absent from our farms and gardens, available only at the grocery store. This was the limit to local food production, my neighbors told me. The prairie of north central Montana was too cold and windy for an orchard. I admitted they might be right. But I wanted to try it for myself.

CHAPTER 10:

Taste of Place

When I was growing up, my family ate a wide variety of local fruit. We had two crab apple trees in our yard, and my grandfather had a plum tree. In the summertime, we looked forward to the wild berries that grew on bushes in our coulees. The first berries to ripen were serviceberries, also called Juneberries, because they matured in late June or early July. Next were the wild currants: black currants, red currants, yellow currants, all of which came on in mid-July. By early August, we could pick chokecherries, which people mostly used for pancake syrup because they had such a strong, astringent flavor. Last were the buffalo berries, which were best after frost. Those were very potent, packed with vitamins and antioxidants. Native people in this area used many of these berries in pemmican—a dried buffalo meat staple that served as the superfood of the northern Great Plains for many generations.

These days, of course, nobody in Big Sandy thinks about local fruit. We just buy stuff at the grocery store that gets shipped here from California or Latin America. I learned just how far removed we've gotten from the idea of growing any of this stuff when I went to the Natural Resources Conservation Service (NRCS) office about a decade ago to see if I could get some advice on how best to set up a water collection system for an orchard. The staff there politely told me that fruit wasn't on their list of crops for our county. It was bureaucratically impossible to grow it here.

Ironically, I actually got more help by venturing farther north—across the Canadian border to the University of Saskatchewan, in Saskatoon. The Canadians knew darn well they couldn't replicate the commercial orchards of temperate Washington or Oregon. So instead of fighting a losing battle to tinker with systems designed for a completely different climate, they looked to their natural surroundings for a better model.

"Take a look at the prairie," one of the Canadian researchers said to me. "Do you see any trees?"

"Not many," I admitted, but there were some cottonwood trees in the creek bottoms, along with the berry bushes that had been the delight of my childhood.

"What two things do those trees have down there in the creek bottoms that are missing on most of the prairie?" the researcher asked. I thought for a minute.

"Shelter. And water."

"Exactly," the researcher said. "So that's what you're going to give your orchard." I could mimic the creek bottoms, he explained, by protecting my trees in the lee of my shelterbelt and setting up a drip irrigation system for summertime.

Encouraged by this conversation, I decided to start my orchard project with something familiar: apples. Given that I'd had them in my yard as a kid, I figured there must be varieties adapted to life on the prairie. I just had to find them. I hunted around our local nurseries and ended up planting thirty varieties of apples, as well as a half dozen different types of plums, four varieties of sour cherries, and two pears. A friend in Missoula helped me select a few grapevine cultivars. Then I added berry bushes: Nanking cherries, gooseberries, elderberries, sand cherries, sea buckthorn—plus some currants, serviceberries, and buffalo berries I dug out of the creek bottom and transplanted. For the first few years, it was all going along pretty well.

Until we had some unusual winters. It started with a very warm autumn—50 or 60 degrees almost up to the end of November. Then, within thirty-six hours, it crashed from 60 degrees to about 8 or 10. Many of my apple trees hadn't yet gone dormant and hardened off because it had been so warm. They were severely damaged by the deep freeze.

The next year we had several chinooks—warm winds in the middle of the winter. Again, the temperature rose to 50 or 60 degrees, sometimes for a week or so. Some of my trees thought it was spring. They started transpiration, so they were losing water to the atmosphere. Meanwhile, the ground was still frozen, so they couldn't get any water from their roots, and they started drying out. Some of them started to break dormancy, and that was the same story as the previous year—when the temperature suddenly plummeted again, they were damaged. Badly. I lost a lot of trees after those two winters. If anyone doubts that climate change is throwing a monkey wrench into farming, they should try growing fruit in Montana.

I needed some advice, so I called up St. Lawrence Nurseries in upstate New York, a place well versed in the trials and tribulations of extreme winters. After a few tries, I managed to reach Bill MacKentley, who had been running the nursery with his wife, Diana, since 1981. In the gravelly voice of an old-timer, Bill poured forth his admiration for the resilient fruit trees of northern climates, which he spoke of as dear friends.

When I told Bill about the difficulties my trees had been having, he asked me something I didn't expect. He wanted to know what rootstock I was using. I was surprised by the question because it looked like the tops of my trees were dying, not the roots. Besides, nearly all the nurseries in our area were selling the same kind of rootstock: semi-dwarf.

The top of the tree—the part that determined what kind of fruit you'd get—was grafted onto the bottom of a different tree, which determined how the tree managed its resources and, thus, how tall it grew. Trees grafted onto semi-dwarf rootstocks, like the ones I'd planted, were popular because they took up less space in backyards and made harvesting fruit a lot easier. No ladders.

But, according to Bill, semi-dwarf trees are always slightly under stress—it comes with the territory of producing more fruit on a slightly smaller plant. In California or North Carolina, this is fine. But in Big Sandy, which is a stressful place for a fruit tree to produce anyway, the added stress of trying to do it with short stature could be fatal.

Given my experience with wheat, I thought I'd learned my lesson about manipulating genetics to maximize production. Something is always compromised. It was the same with the "dilution effect" I'd learned about through my dryland vegetable experiment—higher yields meant lower nutrient density. But this fruit tree thing caught me completely off guard. In all those transactions I'd had with nurseries, no one had ever told me about the Achilles' heel of semi-dwarf trees. We had treated them like some free miracle.

After those two severe winters, I replaced over half of my fruit trees. I got them all from St. Lawrence Nurseries, all standard height. Now I could start thinking about what to do with the harvest.

One of my hardiest fruit crops was the sour cherries. As their name implies, these cherries are pucker-inducing tart—not the kind you would eat fresh but the kind you might use in a pie. Or maybe a breakfast drink. It occurred to me one day, what if we combined the juice from these cherries—which is very nutritious and high in antioxidants but not very sweet—with the juice from our apples, which is also nutritious but almost too sweet to drink straight. Then we would have a breakfast drink from the northern climates, for the northern climates, which I think would be a great substitute for orange juice. Why are we drinking orange juice every morning when there's not an orange tree within a thousand miles of Montana?

The sour cherry and apple breakfast drink isn't on the market yet, but we're already dreaming up additional ways to make the most of local fruit. My oldest daughter, Allison—a natural health enthusiast who makes her own herbal medicines—has taken this on as a project and started experimenting in her kitchen. She lives just up the road in Havre, where her husband practices naturopathic medicine and she gives lectures on healthy and organic cooking at the local natural foods store. So every few weeks, she drops by with some new concoction she's created from the fruits of my orchard.

She started by taking the Concord grapes and making red wine vinegar. I was skeptical of the idea at first, but now I'm hooked—we use it on our salads in place of balsamic. Since then, she's been experimenting with plum vinegar (respectable), pear vinegar (less interesting), the old standard apple vinegar (boring), even currant vinegar (don't even ask; we won't repeat that one). I thought she'd maybe gone too far when she started making sour cherry vinegar, but that turned out to be just as much of a winner as her initial foray with Concord grapes. There are so many opportunities right here in our front yard, literally growing on trees (and in some cases vines and bushes).

I have nothing against orange juice or balsamic vinegar, but what I like about drinking sour cherry and apple juice at breakfast and dressing my salads with my daughter's sour cherry vinegar is that they come from home. These products support our local economy and ecology. And they have a taste that's distinctively Big Sandy.

Celebrating the "taste of place" is typically associated with the French, who coined the term *terroir* ("the flavor or odor of certain locales that are given to its products"), and with wine. In the mid-1850s, the wine producers of Bordeaux became the first vintners to promote the quality of their wares as a function of their place of origin.[1] In 1905, the Champagne region took this focus on geographic indication one step further, passing a law to ensure that its trademark sparkling wine could not be produced elsewhere and marketed under the same name.[2] Much can be learned from the French embrace of a regional food culture, and I think it's worth noting that as American family farms went broke and were bought out in the mid-twentieth century, French farms kept plugging along. As chef and food scholar Amy Trubek observes in her book *Taste of Place*, the share of French farms in the midsize category—between 5 and 50 hectares (12.4–124 acres)—actually *increased* between 1929 and 1983.[3]

But there's nothing exclusively French about regional cuisine. Around the world, people have fashioned culinary traditions from the ingredients around them, blending economic necessity and local pride into foodstuffs symbolic of their origins. North India, which has a temperate climate, developed dishes that utilize wheat and mustard-based spice blends. South India, which is more tropical, leans more heavily on rice and coconut.[4] The cuisine of Japan, an island nation, features fish and seaweed. Thankfully, many of these regional food traditions have refused to give in to the commodity mindset, as cultural ties preserve a sense of common cause connecting farmers, fishers, and eaters committed to the long-term health of their community and its natural resources.

Similar traditions exist among the indigenous peoples of the United States, where buffalo-based foods anchor a sense of place for many of my native neighbors and wild rice plays a large role in the cuisine and environmental ethic of the Ojibwe, six hundred miles to our east in Minnesota. But most people in the United States are relatively recent immigrants. Many of our family food traditions have been lost along the way or inherited from countries with drastically different environmental circumstances. So connecting these food traditions to our place is not always easy. As a result, many food scholars argue, Americans have been particularly susceptible to the rise of cheap commodity foods.

In place of terroir, Americans have tended to embrace the theory of comparative advantage, the philosophical underpinning of globalization and free trade first put forth by economist David Ricardo in the early nineteenth century. The idea of comparative advantage is that it is economically efficient for each country to specialize in what it can produce most cheaply and then trade with other countries to spread cheap goods around to everyone. That is the theory, anyway, but that's not how it tends to work in practice.

In practice, the benefits of comparative advantage accrue not so much to everyday consumers but to large corporations. By shopping around the global marketplace, these corporations end up saving money in multiple ways: first, through lower input and labor costs, and second, through sweetheart deals from governments that have to compete to attract their business. Such deals can include tax incentives, infrastructure, or even exemptions from following the law.

Meanwhile, the free trade system that is supposed to create comparative *advantage* puts downward pressure on the incomes of producers, many of them farmers, who end up being pitted against their counterparts around the world for the lowest cost of production. Free trade economists like to talk about comparative advantages arising from differences in various countries' "natural endowments": climate, terrain, soil type. But in practice, countries often gain comparative advantage through aggressive policies—lower wages, lower environmental standards, and subsidies. As countries compete to be more exploitative of their working people and their environment, the biggest benefits flow to multinational mega-firms, which benefit from a lower cost of doing business.[5] It's a classic race to the bottom.

All of this was painfully familiar to me as a grain farmer. I knew what America's comparative advantage in grain production looked like from my vantage point on the tractor seat: getting paid a pittance to grow cheap commodities for export. Since my farm wasn't growing food for me and my community, we were supposed to use our meager incomes to buy our groceries from someone else. In my younger years, I might have concluded that the farmer who grew my expensive supermarket produce was getting the better end of the deal. But by the time I started planting apple trees, I'd come to realize that "comparative advantage" was just as raw a deal for the Latin American farmers of my counter-seasonal fruit and vegetables as it was for my neighbors growing commodity grain. The real value was being skimmed off by corporate buyers, traders, packagers, and retailers way up the chain, who justified their existence by telling us we were all better off for their services. All of this suggested to me that perhaps we should reconsider the value of growing climate-adapted fruit and vegetables in Big Sandy rather than simply declaring that tropical countries "do it better."

To me, the question we should be asking about comparative advantage is, Who do we want to advantage? Do we want to advantage the multinational corporations that use global trade of cheap commodities to extract value from around the world and concentrate it in their own already bursting coffers? Or do we want to recirculate that value within the communities that generate and sustain it?

If the answer is the latter, embracing taste of place makes a lot of sense. It's already done wonders for the agricultural county of Marin, California, where enthusiasm for the distinctive taste of local dairy products has helped preserve family farms and critical open space resources in a rapidly developing area.[6] In Vermont, the terroir of the region's maple syrup is helping conserve smallholder-owned forests.[7] Big Sandy has longer winters than Marin and a shorter supply of capital, infrastructure, and rain than Vermont. But if I do say so myself, we grow some delicious heritage grains, sour cherries, and dry-farmed squash, and our serviceberry pies are hard to beat.

Some of these Big Sandy specialties, like the grains, came here with immigrants. Others of them, like the berries and squash, have been tended by indigenous Montanans for centuries. Like any regional cuisine, this northern plains fare gives you a taste of the dynamic mixture of cultural traditions that continue to take root in tandem with these plants. This is the neat thing about terroir: it's always in the making.

It all comes back to the lesson I learned from traveling with my high school debate team. Wherever you are, that place is what you and your neighbors make it. From one viewpoint, Big Sandy is a dying, economically depressed little town where the only thing you can grow is cheap commodity wheat. But from another viewpoint, it's the perfect place to raise a family and start a small business growing dryland vegetables or making sour cherry breakfast drinks. Or, as I would discover next, pressing high-oleic safflower into cooking oil.

CHAPTER 11:

Recycling Energy

When I started looking at farming from a net value perspective, I suddenly had to get really honest with myself. I couldn't measure my success solely by my production—that was the commodity mindset. Instead, I had to pay equal attention to my consumption. I had gone some distance down this road by switching to whole, organic heritage grain and growing my own locally adapted fruit and dryland vegetables. I no longer used chemical fertilizer or herbicide, and on my dryland farm we had never used irrigation. But I was still a major consumer of a commodity far more destructive than my conventional wheat had ever been: fossil fuel.

Dependence on fossil energy is so rampant in the American food system that it raises the question, Is agriculture in this country truly a productive activity, or a consumptive one? Researchers estimate that it takes 7 to 10 units of fossil energy to produce 1 unit of food energy in the US food system.[1] Much of that energy being gobbled up by our food system is spent beyond the farm gate, in processing, transportation, storage, and preparation.[2] But American farms use a lot of fossil fuel too: on average, US farmers use 2 kilocalories of fossil energy for every 1 kilocalorie of crop energy they harvest.[3] What kind of business model is that?

The reason American agriculture has gotten away with essentially spending more than it earns is that, particularly since World War II, fossil fuel has been artificially cheap. It's been subsidized by our government. And it's been subsidized again by the public, since we get stuck with the consequences of the industry's unpaid environmental costs. Hence, thanks to the burdens we all bear with our taxes and our bodies, fossil energy has been made to appear inexpensive and abundant, leading to its ubiquitous use in our cars, in our industries, in our consumer products—and on our farms.[4] The result is that, for all the claims that American agriculture has been improved and modernized over the course of the past century, our farming systems have actually become less efficient. In 1910, American growers of one of nature's most energy-efficient crops—corn—produced 5.8 units of energy for every 1 unit they used. By 1983, that ratio had dwindled to just 2.5.[5]

How are American farmers spending all this energy? About one-third of the fossil fuel footprint of contemporary US commodity farms can be chalked up to synthetic nitrogen fertilizer. Another third is due to other inputs: mainly pesticides, but also irrigation—it takes a lot of energy to pump water across thousands of acres of farmland.[6] That means two-thirds of the energy problem with American agriculture can be solved by converting to organics and minimizing supplementary water. So far, so good, I told myself—these were changes I'd made to my operation. But what about that last third?

The last third of fossil energy consumption on American farms is, by and large, just as prevalent on organic farms as on conventional ones—if not more so. This is the diesel fuel we put in our tractors.[7]

Running my farm on diesel didn't sit well with me. As a wheat grower, I'd worked hard to get off the commodity treadmill and control more of my own destiny. That's why I'd started the grain business and gone organic—so I could control my input costs and take my crop to market myself, for a price I thought was fair. But so long as I relied on fossil fuel supplied by cartels, my profit margins were still at the mercy of global commodity prices. My farm's dependence on fossil fuel also cut into the other values I was trying to add: environmental regeneration and social benefit. I didn't see much of that in the way multinational petroleum corporations did business. There had to be a better way.

Given that I was a farmer, the most obvious way for me to source alternative fuel was to grow my own. We can raise lots of different oilseed crops on the northern Great Plains. My neighbors have tried sunflower and canola and safflower. So I thought, Why don't we find one of those crops that works well as a biofuel? We can all add it into our rotations; then some local group can get together and build a facility to crush it into a fuel for our tractors. If a bunch of farmers went in on it, it wouldn't be that expensive. And all the money would stay in the community instead of going to some cartel.

I didn't think canola was the way to go. It did great in Canada, just north of us, or to our west, where the influence of the nearby Rocky Mountains made for cooler weather. But here, it would often bloom in the hottest part of the summer and the flowers would be destroyed because they were too fragile to withstand the heat. My neighbors who had grown safflower complained that it matured so late that you had to go get your combine back out of the shed as winter was approaching. It's not uncommon for farmers in my area to pull eighteen-hour days during harvest season in July and August and then hit winter wheat seeding hard in September. By Halloween, we're all ready for a break.

But then came along a brand-new option, a crop being promoted by a researcher at a nearby experiment station. This oilseed crop could be planted in March in very cold soils, which meant it would bloom in June, before the heat came on. It was called camelina.

To see if camelina would like it at my place, I grew a test plot of half an acre. That turned out pretty well, so I scaled up to twenty acres in my second year, and I did another thirty-five acres or so the following year. I had a brief misadventure with my first attempt to press the camelina into oil. It was a good reminder about the real value of cheap goods: I bought a cheap press, and I couldn't get the thing to work at all. As a last-ditch effort, I invited all my best mechanic friends to come over one Saturday morning and help me. By Saturday afternoon, all we had to show for our efforts was a gallon jug of brownish oil that smelled like coffee. Burnt coffee.

So I got a higher-quality oil press, which worked like a dream. My son, thirteen at the time, was able to run it by himself. I had already purchased the other piece of equipment I needed—a digester to convert the pressed camelina oil into biodiesel so we could run it in our tractor. Our homegrown energy experiment was ready to launch! But the more I learned about biodiesel, the more I started having second thoughts.

To convert vegetable oil into biodiesel, you need to use lye. When you wash out the lye, you end up with wastewater—and a by-product, glycerin. I didn't know where I could find a market for high volumes of glycerin. This whole idea wasn't looking quite so closed-loop after all.

Then a friend from the educational farm at the University of Montana came to my rescue. He said I didn't need to make biodiesel. I could use straight vegetable oil. All I had to do was modify my tractor so that it would preheat the vegetable oil to 160 degrees. This would reduce the viscosity of the oil, so it would go into the engine hot and act just like diesel.

The catch was, there were only certain kinds of vegetable oil that could go straight into a tractor. Camelina oil was *poly*unsaturated, meaning the long fatty acid chains in each molecule had multiple double carbon bonds. From a chemical standpoint, those multiple double bonds made the camelina oil susceptible to oxidation, which meant it could gunk up my engine and rapidly go rancid in storage. What I needed was an oil that was *mono*unsaturated—just one double carbon bond. That's when I learned about high-oleic safflower.

I'd never thought much about the balance of fats in a safflower seed. As far as I knew, the main market for safflower was birdseed, and I didn't think the birds were all that picky about types of fat. But what might not matter to the birds was critically important for my tractor, my friend from UM told me.

Most of the safflower grown for birdseed, my friend explained, is high in *linoleic* acid—a polyunsaturated fatty acid, similar to those found in camelina. But there were other varieties of safflower bred to be high in *oleic* acid, which had the monounsaturated fat I was looking for.

Figuring I'd found the solution to my fuel problem, I sold my digester and planted forty acres of high-oleic safflower. (The unused camelina seed went to a chicken feed outfit in Washington, and a natural food retailer in Boston bought the camelina oil I had already pressed.) That first crop made me really nervous, because it took so long to mature. I was used to wheat and barley, fast-growing grains that cover the field within just a few weeks of planting. Not safflower. It took its time. But once it started to bloom, oh my goodness. The field was a glistening sea of golden yellow blossoms, which turned to orange as the crop ripened. I walked into the rows of flowering energy factories to check on their progress toward harvest and was immediately checked by the sensation of little pins pricking me. The safflower had grown stickers everywhere, all over the leaves and even the flowers. It was like a thistle. I had another surprise as we harvested the crop, when the air conditioner in my combine suddenly quit working. Inside the seed heads of the safflower, I discovered, were large quantities of very fine fibers—which were plugging up the air conditioner's filters. They shut it right down. But once I learned to clean the air filters every day and wear heavy gloves and leather chaps in the field, I found safflower quite an agreeable crop.

Yes, it meant a little bit longer season, but the plants produced well, and the seeds were readily converted to oil in the press we'd purchased for camelina. Now all I had to do was convert my tractor, and I was ready to run my farm on homegrown fuel.

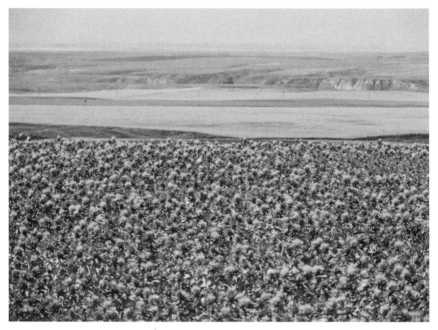

SAFFLOWER FIELD IN LATE BLOOM WITH THE MISSOURI RIVER BREAKS
IN THE BACKGROUND.
(Photo by Hilary Page)

Then my hired man threw me a curveball. He took some of my high-oleic safflower oil to one of the restaurants in Big Sandy. They tried using it as cooking oil and loved it. The restaurant owner asked if we would consider selling to him and said he'd be willing to pay us nearly $2 per pound. I did the math and determined that was almost $16 per gallon. And I was getting ready to pour this oil into my tractor to replace diesel fuel, which cost about one-fourth as much. Now I had a genuine sustainability dilemma on my hands. I knew the best decision for our business was to sell the oil to restaurants. But I didn't want to give up on my original goal of replacing fossil fuel with something homegrown and renewable. This was the frustration I found myself confessing to Ian Finch, director of sustainability for University of Montana Dining Services.

Ian had been up to my farm before, as part of a UM field course that often visited us in the summer, so he knew all about the ancient wheat and the dryland vegetables. But he was surprised to hear I was now growing safflower—and he wanted to know more. In 2012, we arranged a meeting at his office in the University Center at UM. Sitting around the table were me, Ian, and my son-in-law Andrew Long, who had recently moved back to the farm with my youngest daughter, Bridgette, to run the oil business. I had offered Andrew the job right out of his MBA, thinking we could use some help with our launch and he could use the experience on his résumé. I'd asked Andrew for only a one-year commitment, figuring he might want to move on to one of the big-city jobs he'd trained for. But after a year, he told me he was having more fun than any of his classmates—so he and Bridgette settled in right next door to me, in the house my folks vacated when they went into assisted living in Great Falls. Andrew was a sharp guy, and he was just as interested as I was in building a creative partnership with the University of Montana.

UM Dining relied on large quantities of vegetable oil to serve the campus thousands of meals per day, Ian told Andrew and me. They had been using a blended product from a plant in northeastern Montana, but that plant had recently closed. It wasn't hard to see the flaw in the business model. This plant had been extracting oil from oilseeds using hexane—to get the very last drop of oil out of the seed. They maximized the production, all right, but the result was that their mash became a toxic waste product. You couldn't even feed it to animals. They ruined their by-product trying to squeeze the last little bit of marginal value out of the first product. They were in a race to the bottom, always competing with cheaper and cheaper oils, from larger and larger plants. Textbook value subtraction commodity mindset.

When this conventional vegetable oil plant shut down, UM Dining went looking for another Montana supplier, which is why they called me. The campus already had a Farm-to-College program, which was Ian's domain, and they were committed to sourcing in-state and sustainably whenever possible. But our cost of production was higher than that of the conventional plant, which meant our prices were higher too. The conventional plant, like most cooking oil manufacturers, had mixed together whatever vegetable oils it could source most cheaply and covered up any shortfalls in quality with a host of additives. In contrast, we were using organically grown high-oleic safflower, which was more expensive. And, of course, we hadn't yet decided to go into the culinary oil market, anyway.

"How about we just give it a try?" Ian proposed, figuring there was no harm in an experiment. We agreed to drop off thirty-five gallons of our oil so the chefs in UM's various kitchens and cafés could trial it in their recipes. As the trial progressed, the chefs made some remarkable discoveries. The first thing they noticed was that there was less transfer of flavors from one dish to another than they'd had with their conventional oil. If they used high-oleic safflower oil to cook fish and then chicken and then potatoes, they didn't end up with fishy-tasting potatoes. The stability of the oil meant they could use it longer—getting more bang for their buck. Intrigued by this finding, UM ran tests to find out just how long they could use safflower oil before it degraded. They found that the safflower oil held up significantly longer than blended cooking oil products or canola oil—meaning it had not only a longer cooking life but a longer shelf life too. That made sense to me—the whole reason we'd gone with high-oleic safflower was that it was more stable. I was thinking about tractors, not woks, but biochemically, it was the same principle.

The UM chefs loved the flavor of the safflower oil, and they tried all sorts of things with it that I never would have imagined. They fried in it, as they had done with their previous blended oil product. But they also used it for baking, grilling—even as an ingredient in salad dressings. UM had previously stocked different oils to do each of these things, and the overhead associated with all that inventory was adding up. The versatility of safflower oil meant they could cut that inventory by more than half.

But the person who really convinced UM Dining that safflower oil was the way to go was their registered dietitian. While trying to move students away from fried foods, UM Dining had learned that discontinuing these items entirely meant students would just go off campus to get them elsewhere. So UM decided on a pragmatic strategy: if fried foods were a nonnegotiable part of their students' diet, Dining Services wanted to do what it could to make those chicken nuggets and tater tots as healthy as possible. Safflower oil, the dietitian found, was one of the healthiest oils to deep-fat fry in—and our cold-pressed product was free of the TBHQ (tertiary butylhydroquinone) and other chemical ingredients that commodity oil suppliers regularly added to their products as anti-foaming agents and preservatives, despite mounting evidence that these are dangerous to consume in any quantity.[8]

Had UM run a traditional cost-benefit analysis on their safflower oil experiment, they would have concluded that our oil was too expensive. It cost twice as much as canola oil or a blended product, and even the longer cooking life and reduced inventory costs weren't enough to completely make up the difference. But UM didn't run a traditional cost-benefit analysis. They looked at the full spectrum of safflower oil's value: from the crop's role in organic rotations and the rural Montana economy to the long-term health of their students. From that standpoint, safflower oil came out a clear winner. UM asked if we would consider becoming their regular vegetable oil supplier. It was a great opportunity for us, I told Ian, but I was still frustrated about ending up on the wrong side of my fuel versus food dilemma.

Competition between fuel production and food production is a major sustainability concern with biofuels. Normally the worry is that fuel use will trump food use, as has happened with corn ethanol, which has led to croplands being converted to fuel cars instead of feeding people. When we start asking farms to fuel our cities, I think we are inevitably going to run into this problem. In my case, I had a less ambitious goal: using a small part of my farm to fuel just the farm itself. And I was concerned that the UM Dining deal would put me back in the commodity conundrum: exporting something off the farm (a potential energy source) that I would then have to import from someone else (a cartel). On the cusp of achieving a closed-loop fuel solution, I didn't want to sell my energy independence down the river.

Then I had an idea: why not go ahead and sell the oil to UM but recover the waste oil and burn it in my diesel engine? I asked Ian if he might consider such an arrangement.

What if we thought of it as a sort of rental agreement, I proposed. After all, the UM chefs weren't exactly *using* most of the oil. When they cooked in it, they didn't use the oil up; they just employed it to perform a service: transforming raw food into a meal. When it was done performing that service and had degraded beyond its usefulness in the kitchen, it became a liability. A waste product. They had to pay to dispose of it.

So instead of letting all that oil go to waste, I suggested, why not send it back to me and Andrew? UM could return it to my farm in the same containers we delivered it in—transforming their liability (waste oil) into our asset (fuel). We didn't need to choose between fuel value and food value—we could utilize both!

The oil we get back from UM is enough to provide about one-eighth of the fuel needs for our farm, and we're now actively looking for other customers to "rent" the remaining seven-eighths of our homegrown energy en route to the fuel tank. Vegetable oil is not so great as a fuel in the winter because it becomes too viscous in extreme cold. But we don't farm in the winter.

In addition to fuel value and food value, we've added a third source of value to our safflower crop: feed. Because we extract our oil using a cold press at low temperatures instead of hexane, we end up with a mash by-product that is nontoxic and still 3 or 4 percent oil. At 21 percent protein, it makes a good supplementary feed for cattle, and we're now selling it to Organic Valley for their dairy cows.

What this all means is that with high-oleic safflower, we can use our farm production first for food, then for feed, then for fuel. We call this business The Oil Barn, and with my son-in-law now at the helm, we've started making some small retail bottles of the oil too, so people can try it in their homes. Our latest idea is to pair the oil with my daughter Allison's homegrown red wine vinegar as a Montana-made salad dressing.

The Oil Barn is still a pretty modest demonstration, but I think oil-seed crops used first for food and then for fuel could be a viable substitute for at least some of the diesel we use on farms. Infrastructure like the oil press and cleaning equipment we've installed could be purchased by a farmer cooperative, which could serve as both its own supplier and its own customer. Eliminating our dependence on fossil fuel would shield farmers from the worrying ups and downs of diesel prices—and make us much more valuable net contributors to the real wealth of our communities and our planet.

Of course, farmers aren't the only ones worried about dependence on fossil fuels. I've had a number of urban people ask me if I think the Oil Barn model could provide sustainable fuel for their vehicles. But at that scale, I think the closed loop breaks down. As we've seen with most large-scale experiments with biofuels, importing huge quantities of energy from the countryside to our urban centers overtaxes land and

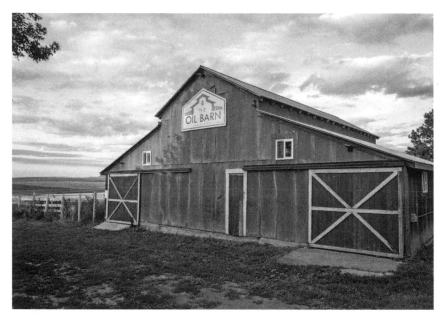

THE OIL BARN MANUFACTURING FACILITY, IN MY RENOVATED COW BARN.
(Photo by Jamen Long)

rural communities. It's not as environmentally destructive as fossil fuel development, but it's still extractive—and it can displace food crops. So I don't think we should try to have farmers grow all the energy for cities. For cities, we need to tap into other renewable resources, like solar and wind. But farmers can help with that too—because if you've ever been to north central Montana farm country, you know that we are very rich in wind.

In 1999, I traveled to Germany to research my family history, and while I was there, I went to visit a place where some of my ancestors had lived hundreds of years ago. It was a castle, and the guy I found living there still carried the title of a nobleman: *Graf*, which is the German equivalent of "count." According to my research, he was my fourteenth cousin twice removed.

I was a bit intimidated to introduce myself to the Graf, whose ascot tie and precisely tailored pants hinted at his social standing. But the dapper, wiry nobleman was surprisingly genial and invited me in to chat. When I told the Graf I was interested in family history, he took me down a hallway where a three- by four-foot chart was posted in an old, ornate frame, documenting centuries of the family lineage. My line had broken off from his way up at the top, but there it was, still preserved behind the glass. Just down the hall were giant portraits, some even bigger than the chart, depicting the castle's previous inhabitants. It was like stepping back in time.

Except, that is, for the conspicuously modern-looking wind turbines on the property. When I inquired about them, the Graf asked me if I might like to climb one. What the heck, I thought. We walked to the base of one of the turbines, which looked bigger up close: somewhere in the neighborhood of one hundred fifty to two hundred feet tall. The Graf unlocked the door to the central column and flipped a switch. Almost instantly, the blades stopped spinning. "Put this on," the Graf said, handing me a harness. Once we were strapped in, we began climbing a ladder, up, up, up the central column until we finally reached the top of the turbine. Winded, I stopped for a moment to catch my breath. Now standing just feet from the generator of the mighty energy machine, I felt a jolt as the Graf switched the turbine back on. The wind wasn't particularly strong that day, but I was perched right in front of the turbine's blades now, and I could see that they were turning at a decent clip. "Hang on," the Graf said, flipping the switch again to turn the turbine off. Again, the blades came to a halt almost immediately— with such force that they jolted the whole platform to one side. This was powerful stuff, I thought.

Once we were safely back on terra firma, the Graf told me that he and his business partner were building wind farms, starting at his place and then expanding to other places in the world. They'd started a company called Wind Park Solutions, and they were thinking about putting turbines in South Africa, Chile, and Argentina.

You don't have to go that far, I told the Graf. The last time the wind stopped blowing in our neighborhood, half the buildings fell down. My corny Big Sandy joke got the Graf chuckling but also seriously thinking about the possibility. Within three months, he was on a plane to Montana with his business partner, eager to find a suitable site for a wind farm.

Before they arrived, the Graf told me about his business partner's uncanny knack for finding the best locations for turbines. "He observes the trees," the Graf told me. "He can read their growth habits like a weather vane." There was just one problem with that, I told the Graf. On the prairie, there are no trees—except along the riverbeds and in some shelterbelts that farmers have planted. Having never seen the American Great Plains, the Graf was perplexed. No trees? What sort of place was this?

We didn't need to observe trees to find our wind farm site, though. About a hundred miles due south from my house, near the little town of Judith Gap, there was a sign along the highway that read "Danger: High Wind Area." Next to it was a wind sock so you could see just how windy it was as you attempted to keep your truck on the road. I'd driven by that sign probably a dozen times without ever realizing what it was trying to tell me: build your wind farm right here! When I took the German guys down to Judith Gap, they methodically set up towers to monitor the wind to tell us the potential of that site. Their measurements told us what everybody in Judith Gap already knew: it was really windy.

We had plenty of wind. We had a new company, Wind Park Solutions America. What we didn't have were state regulations that spelled out how to permit a wind farm. Montana had never had one before.

Although I didn't have a history in the energy business, I knew the typical playbook well enough from watching the coal and oil developers who frequently proposed projects in our state. As far as I could tell, their goal was to permit their projects as quickly as they could, with as little involvement from regulatory agencies and the public as possible. Given that their objective appeared to be to extract near-term value, that was probably a logical approach.

But our objective was different: we wanted to create long-term, regenerative value. In our minds, Judith Gap was just the beginning. On the horizon were other wind farms, and perhaps solar and geothermal projects: a future of renewable energy for the northern Great Plains. We didn't plan to develop all these projects ourselves, but they were part and parcel of our vision. Our goal wasn't just to be the first wind farm in Montana. Our goal was to make sure we weren't the last wind farm in Montana.

So we used the opposite playbook: we put our plans out in the open and spent three years actively soliciting public scrutiny and regulatory input. We talked to the people of Judith Gap, the county commissioners in nearby Harlowton, the regulatory agencies in Helena who dealt with energy and environment, the community of environmental scientists who had expertise or concerns about wind turbines. We held public meetings. We conducted environmental impact studies. We met with state legislators and other elected officials to figure out how to make the permitting process work for everyone.

Concerns about the project fell into two categories. On the one hand, some environmental groups were worried that our wind turbines might kill birds. This had been a problem with some of the first-generation wind turbines built in California with insufficient attention to migratory flight patterns. We didn't want to make the same mistake in Montana, so we commissioned studies of bird traffic, both by day (which could be observed easily enough) and by night (which required radar). We chose a spot that didn't appear to be in a major flight path and then went looking for bird studies conducted by other wind farms to see if we could find any that had a comparable level of bird traffic. As luck would have it, we found two bird-abundance-comparable wind farms, both of which had been built and had kept records of bird mortality. Based on these analogous wind farms, we estimated that each of our turbines would kill one or two birds per year—far fewer than a typical automobile or house cat.

On the other hand, we met with significant opposition from the coal industry, which saw that if Montanans were allowed to harvest the wind, they might not buy so much fossil energy. But the coal lobby had trouble casting themselves as defenders of Montanans' best interests, because we did extensive surveys of local people in Judith Gap and the surrounding region, who had no doubt that renewable energy was a good deal for them. As of the 2000 census, more than one-third of the population of Judith Gap had been living below the poverty line. This wind farm was an opportunity to bring significant income to the county through taxes, and unlike fossil fuel energy, it wouldn't come with environmental damage. Not surprisingly, local enthusiasm for the project was high: 15 percent of the population of Wheatland County filled out a survey about the wind farm, and all respondents but one were in favor.[9]

With the community in support and the environmental impact studies on file, Montana was ready to move forward with its first wind farm. The Montana Power Company put out a request for proposals, and we submitted our plan for Judith Gap.

We came in second.

We were disappointed, but it turned out that the guy who came in first had made up some things, and the winning proposal wasn't actually a viable one. So Montana Power repeated the whole process, and this time we came in first.

Just as we thought construction might be moving forward, Montana Power began restructuring into a telecommunications company (a complete boondoggle) and sold off its power operations to NorthWestern Energy. *They* had to do the proposal process a third time. We won again, and finally, it looked like we had a green light.

But because the guy who won the first round had submitted unreliable information, NorthWestern Energy required that the wind farm be built and operated by a company that had experience and had successfully done a similar project before, in the United States. I was a first-timer, and my business partner was German. So we had to sell the project to a developer who built it and made the lion's share of the money.

That was fine by us, though, because we achieved all our goals.

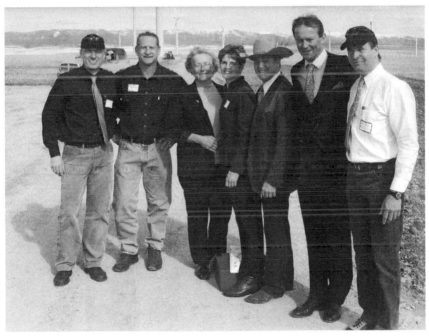

OCTOBER 2005 DEDICATION OF WIND PARK SOLUTIONS AMERICA (WPSA) IN JUDITH GAP, MONTANA'S FIRST WIND FARM. FROM LEFT TO RIGHT: STEFFEN CHUN (WPSA); DAVE RYAN (NORTHWESTERN ENERGY); WENDY KLEINSASSER (WPSA); MY WIFE, ANN, AND ME; GEORG VON WEDEL, "THE GRAF" (WPSA); JOERG BELAND (WPSA).
(Photo by Mo Scarpelli)

Montana got its first commercial-scale wind farm, at 135 megawatts, in October 2005.[10] The Judith Gap turbines supplied energy to 30,000 homes per year, generating a dozen jobs and $1.2 million in annual tax revenue for economically struggling Wheatland County without raising utility bills or harming the environment.[11] And, as we'd vowed, Montana's first wind farm wasn't its last. From 2005 to 2015, 60 percent of new energy capacity constructed in Montana was wind power.[12]

For a state that's done a lot of choking on coal dust and refinery smoke—with most of the profits extracted out of our communities along with our natural resources—wind energy is a very positive development. We're so used to thinking of energy development as extractive that it's hard to imagine it as a potentially regenerative activity—something that might actually help us *heal* rural areas battered by the boom-and-bust cycles of coal and oil. But in Montana, we're already moving toward that future, with surprising buy-in across the political spectrum.

CHAPTER 12:

Bringing Rural Jobs Back

Grain. Vegetables. Fruit. Energy. I was starting to sketch out a blueprint for the future of Big Sandy and the revitalization of rural America. But I still had one piece of unfinished business. I couldn't stop thinking about Corn Nuts.

Way back in the 1970s, that had been my first business idea: to take our "King Tut's wheat"—as we called it at the time—and make it into a snack. If it worked with giant corn, it ought to work with giant wheat. I still thought it was a good idea.

Corn Nuts, however, had long since been bought by Mars, Incorporated. Good luck trying to get on the phone with someone in product development there. I may as well have been attempting to reach the pope. I tried to interest a few other companies in the idea, but nobody picked it up.

Remember how I said I would never go into the food-manufacturing business? That I was going to stick to what I do best—farming—and find partners with the know-how to take the product into the test kitchen? I guess I should never say never. I really wanted to try a Kamut-based version of Corn Nuts. And it appeared the only way to do it was to make it myself.

It wasn't lost on me, of course, that if this snack took off, I could create jobs in my local community of Big Sandy. Vertically integrating my business—from the grain production all the way through to the finished food—meant all the value would circulate here. I had a vision of people going to minor league baseball games in Great Falls and enjoying a snack that was grown, cooked, and packaged by their neighbors.

I started out by working with one of *my* neighbors, who experimented with small batches of a Kamut snack in her kitchen. She boiled the seed, let it dry slightly, then fried it in our high-oleic safflower oil. I thought it tasted pretty good, and I told her we should make more.

My neighbor's nephew managed a combination bowling alley and restaurant that had big fryers, so we went over there to do our first large-scale production run. We were a crew of five: my wife and me, my neighbor and her husband, plus their nephew—who told us we could get started just as soon as the restaurant closed. That turned out to be pretty late at night, and my wife and I finally had to bow out at two in the morning. But the other three kept going until daybreak and got the job done.

The next day, we brought the Kamut snacks back to my house in big buckets and started packaging them by hand around the kitchen table. We had arranged to sell our first batch at one of those minor league baseball games in Great Falls. My oldest daughter came over with her kids to help package, and she sampled a little bit of the snack to see what she thought.

"Dad, this is terrible," my daughter told me. "Only half the kernels are crispy, and the other half are hard as a rock."

I tried some myself. My daughter was right. It turned out that our wee-hours crew had gotten ahead on the cooking and behind on the frying, and some of the grain had dried out too much in between. They didn't realize it at the time, so everything had gotten mixed together.

We never sold any Kamut snacks at that ball game. Just as I'd feared, vertical integration was harder than it looked, and my neighbors weren't up for any more late night production runs. I wasn't ready to give up yet, though, so I started nosing around for a bright young person who might be interested in moving to Big Sandy and doing some mad Kamut science in a makeshift test kitchen.

I found one. His name was Caleb Kriser, and he was just finishing up an undergraduate degree in Idaho, studying agricultural business. I hired him right out of school, and he immediately set up shop in my shed. For over a year, Caleb made Kamut snacks out there in the shed, refining the cooking and the soaking process until it was ready for prime time. In a complete stroke of luck, we found a company just north of us in Canada that had been making a similar product but was getting out of the snack business. They offered to sell us all their machinery at a very reasonable cost.

Just as we were about to close the deal with the company in Canada, the person who had signed on to help me with that year's harvest pulled out at the last minute. So I had to take Caleb off the Kamut snack project for three months to fill in. By the time all the crops were in the bin in September, the people in Canada were no longer interested in selling us their equipment. They were no longer confident we were serious, and since the deal involved paying them off with a share of our profits, they were worried they'd never see the money if we didn't get our business off the ground.

This put us in a real bind. As Caleb searched the internet for another source of equipment, we found two sizes: kitchen size and industrial size. And when I say industrial size, I mean *large* industrial size. Gargantuan.

We were a small business, looking to produce our snacks on a medium scale. We weren't Mars. But we weren't home cooks either. And just as I'd found years earlier with my grain mill, the whole American food system has a yawning gap in the middle. It seemed there wasn't a single company building commercial kitchen equipment with businesses of our scale in mind.

Eventually, we found a solution overseas. In China, they have these small batch fryers that are about a meter or so in diameter and handle about thirty or forty pounds in a batch. That was perfect for us. We got our shipment from China, and while it wasn't plug and play, Caleb got it going without too much trouble.

By June 2015, we were ready to officially open the doors of Big Sandy Organics and debut our Kracklin' Kamut snacks. I planned the grand opening to coincide with the homecoming celebration that Big Sandy High School holds every five years for all its alumni. It's old home week for proud Big Sandy natives, doubling the population of the town for the weekend, so I thought it would be the perfect time to welcome the community to check out our new enterprise and try the snacks.

Then my dad died.

My father was nearly ninety-four years old and suffering from dementia, so his death wasn't a complete surprise. But just five years earlier, he'd driven my combine for me for half a day, and we'd had a good visit just hours before he passed. It seemed fitting that he should be here to see the full circle of this crop he had found for me in his friend's basement, this crop that he had insisted on taking to the natural food show in California, where he found our first customer. It was my dad who'd been there on the other end of the phone four decades earlier when I'd first cooked up my harebrained scheme to talk Corn Nuts into making snacks out of a giant wheat. It was my dad who'd painstakingly grown it out. And it was my dad who'd held onto the seed—and the dream—when our first deal fell through. I had a speech all prepared to give him the credit he was due when that dream finally became a reality and our factory doors opened to the public. But now he wouldn't be here to hear it.

It was with mixed feelings and a heavy heart that I celebrated our grand opening that Friday, as I prepared for my dad's funeral the following Monday. But as people poured into our little facility—some from across the street, others from across the state—the excitement was palpable. We'd all had enough of seeing rural businesses close their doors. It was a lot more gratifying to open them.

We started selling Kracklin' Kamut snacks at some of the local grocery stores and gas stations. A few of the bars on Big Sandy's Main Street bought some to provide to their patrons. Our local 4-H chapter sold some as a fund-raiser, and then the snacks got picked up by a handful of Future Farmers of America groups around the state for the same purpose. It was a totally different market from the artisanal pasta and the wheatgrass drinks. I loved it.

With the help of a friend from the food show circuit, I designed the original bag for the snack. I had in mind the Fort Benton County Fair, where I had first seen the ancient wheat the snack was made out of and where some of the first bags were sold by our local 4-H kids. I imagined fairgoers putting this snack in their pocket along with a handful of carnival ride tickets. I imagined it at the ball games. I wanted it to be fun. So I insisted we make the package bright and shiny, with colorful reds and oranges. I'm not interested in building an *alternative* market anymore. I think real food grown without chemicals should be for everyone.

A longtime organic farmer from Missoula came up for a visit while I was working on the Kracklin' Kamut package design, and I asked him what he thought. "Bob," he told me, "that doesn't look very organic." Dang, I thought. Nailed it.

Caleb eventually decided to move on, but I was able to replace him with another bright young tinkerer, Thomas Dilworth, who is now the plant manager of Big Sandy Organics. Then Thomas connected me with a childhood friend of his who is a wizard of an engineer and has helped us trick out our new facility, which we opened in the summer of 2017. The mail-order cooking apparatus from China got us started, but it had some glitches, like when the boiler started spitting fire. So Thomas and his friend have helped us replace all that with custom equipment made in the United States.

Now you can buy Kracklin' Kamut snacks at grocery stores across the region. We see that there's room for growth, and just like my childhood batches of ice cream, it's a fun thing to be able to share with the neighbors.

But the best thing about vertically integrating this business in Big Sandy is that every job we create really matters. This is rural America, where the poverty rate is nearly four percentage points higher than in urban areas.[1] While the urban job market has recovered from the 2008 recession—there are now 4 percent *more* metropolitan jobs available than there were in 2008—the rural job market is 4.26 percent smaller.[2] The frustrations connected to this poverty of opportunity have ugly consequences, among them a staggering opioid epidemic that threatens to turn temporary unemployment into permanent unemployment for many rural people. Those who are working—mostly farmers—are under tremendous strain from struggling to earn a living in the cheap food economy. Suicide rates for Americans working in agriculture are among the highest in the nation, higher even than those reported for military veterans.[3]

The key to breaking this cycle of decline and despair, I think, is to make sure everyone has the opportunity to work a stable, meaningful, well-paying job. I'm proud to have created a few such opportunities: The staff at Montana Flour and Grains in Fort Benton has now grown to fourteen, and four Montanans work for Kamut International, along with our staff in Europe. My farm has five employees—and there are two people working at The Oil Barn.

Big Sandy Organics is just in its infancy, with two full-time employees and some high school students part-time. But I think we can grow this business to the point that it will be a significant employer in Big

Sandy and make a difference to our local economy. In a small town, it doesn't take much.

Currently, I have a total of nine employees in Big Sandy, between the Kracklin' Kamut project and The Oil Barn and my farm. Those nine employees have a total of 18 kids among them. So in a school system that has approximately 120 kids, that's an addition of 15 percent. Sometimes that can be the difference between keeping the school's doors open and closing it down.

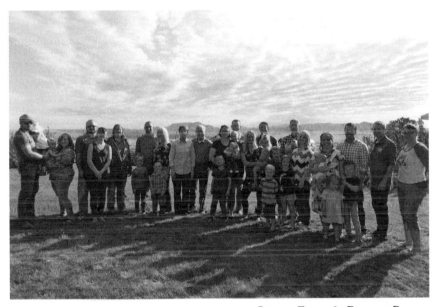

THE PEOPLE WHO MAKE IT ALL HAPPEN AT QUINN FARM & RANCH, BIG SANDY ORGANICS, AND THE OIL BARN, IN BIG SANDY WITH THEIR FAMILIES. (Photo by Hilary Page)

Nine jobs (or ten, if I count myself) is good, but my goal is to create twelve. Back in my grandparents' generation, a homestead was 320 acres. My farm is 4,000 acres, roughly twelve homesteads. So in order to bring back the neighbors that we've lost to "get big or get out" agriculture, I figure our farm and our value-added enterprises need to support twelve families. If we get an airline to pick up our Kracklin' Kamut snacks, I think we might get there in the next couple of years.

It's not that I'm some brilliant entrepreneur or anything like that. Everywhere you have organic agriculture, you have these kinds of stories—because it's a business that's fundamentally based on adding and regenerating value, not extracting it. In 2016, the Organic Trade Association commissioned a study on the link between organics and economic development.[4] Edward C. Jaenicke, a professor of agricultural economics at Pennsylvania State University, conducted the study, which came to be known as the "organic hotspots report." Professor Jaenicke identified 225 US counties that had high levels of organic agricultural activity and also neighbored counties with high levels of organic agricultural activity. These were the hotspots. Then he looked at census data to see how these counties were faring economically. Jaenicke concluded that being an organic hotspot increases median household incomes by over $2,000 and reduces county poverty rates by as much as 1.35 percent.

Jaenicke also made another important finding: although high levels of *organic* agricultural activity led to economic advantages, high levels of *non-organic* agricultural activity did not. This might seem surprising, given the truly astonishing levels of farm production coming out of our nation's chemical agriculture hotspots. It stands to reason that farmers and farm communities should benefit from this bounty. But by and large, they don't. Rather, it's just as the US Department of Agriculture's Walter Goldschmidt warned us back in the 1940s with his landmark study of California's rapidly industrializing agriculture. The bigger and more industrial the farms, the poorer and less vibrant the rural communities.[5]

The seven-decade experiment with chemically supported farming that we ironically call conventional (although it is completely out of step with the conventions that farmers have followed for most of the ten thousand years of human agricultural history) is not adding value for farmers. The chemical industry sells farmers expensive inputs based on the premise that the inputs will boost farmers' yields, and they let the farmers assume that higher yields will translate into a lot of money. What they don't talk about is the cost of producing those yields—and sometimes the costs are higher than the returns.

When I started farming my grain organically, I dramatically lowered the cost I paid for my inputs. At the same time, I increased the value of what I sold. Maybe the yields were a little bit less, although they can be pretty competitive in a dry year. But I still came out way ahead. Depending on the weather, the net is 30 to 50 to 100 percent greater than what my chemical neighbors get, even in average market conditions. And in a year like 2017, when commodity wheat prices were low, net returns on organic grain can be as much as three times as high as conventional. Best of all, I don't have to take out an operating loan, so I don't owe interest to the bank.

Some people say organic food is not as economically efficient because it requires more management, more labor. But I don't look at it as more labor; I look at it as more jobs.[6] If you have increased your net profits to the point where you can afford to hire people from your local community, I say that's a win-win. I would much rather put a dollar in my neighbor's pocket than send another dollar off to Monsanto.

It was this dimension of value—dollars and cents—that had inspired me to go into business in the first place, and all these years later, I was still primarily focused on economic development for rural America. Along the way, though, I'd learned that adding real value to our local economy had an environmental dimension as well, which was crucial to the long-term sustainability of the community's bottom line. This environmental dimension of value wasn't always acknowledged in business circles, but I came to believe it should be—and I had become a passionate advocate for fundamentally greening our economy. Increasingly, I was starting to see that another critically important dimension of my community's bottom line was also being left out of business discussions and completely neglected by the mainstream food system. Health. It was time to put my researcher hat back on and finally answer some of my nagging questions about what our diets were doing to our bodies.

CHAPTER 13:

The Gluten Mystery

In 2000, a naturopathic doctor named Rossana Marrella stopped by our Kamut booth at a natural food show in Italy. A compact woman with gestures that rivaled the size of her body, Rossana spoke passionately about her frustration with the pill-pushing approach of mainstream medicine and her determination to get to the bottom of her patients' health issues. She'd been studying a problem she didn't fully understand, and she wondered if we knew of any research on the matter.

"People keep coming to see me with some symptom or another related to eating wheat," Rossana told us. "But when they switch to an ancient grain, most of their symptoms go away. I know there's something different about how the older wheats interact with the digestive system. But I don't know precisely what it is."

Ever since our family friend with environmental sensitivities had told my father that Kamut pasta made her feel better, I had been looking for researchers who might want to collaborate with me on nutritional studies of ancient grain. As a researcher myself, I had often turned to agronomic scientists to help me resolve questions about my farm, and once I began to see the connections between farming and health, I felt I ought to be consulting with nutritionists as well. But for the most part, I struck out. Wheat is wheat, I was told. It all has gluten, so why would ancient wheat be any different? It wasn't that the scientists I spoke with had ethical concerns about working with a grower who might benefit from their findings. If they had, I could have respected that. Ideally, funding for nutritional studies would come from sources that didn't have skin in the game.

But unfortunately, much of the financial backing for nutrition science in the United States comes from big players in agribusiness. Heavily invested in modern wheat, these corporate funders weren't terribly interested in supporting science that could call their products' nutritional value into question. To the contrary—they worked back-channel connections to influence not only privately funded science but also government dietary regulations.[1] In this environment, it was risky for American researchers to take self-reported "gluten sensitivity" seriously and investigate whether there might actually be something wrong with modern grain varieties. So the differences between ancient and modern grains garnered little scientific attention, and instead of reforming wheat, Americans gradually abandoned it. Each year when I wandered the aisles of Natural Products Expo West, I saw ever-growing quantities of rice pasta and potato flour bread. "Wheat free" and "gluten free" were everywhere.

Italians, as I'd learned from my visits to Europe, were more stubborn. Their food culture told them that wheat had been in their diet for generations, and it belonged there. They went looking for wheat they could eat and eventually found their way to older varieties. By the late 1990s, Rossana was one among many health professionals recommending ancient grain to patients who told her they were gluten sensitive or had the characteristic symptoms. But she was troubled by how little she and her colleagues actually knew about why this prescription seemed to work.

By this point, researchers had already established many health benefits of *whole* grains. Epidemiological studies—surveys of large populations that analyze relationships between health outcomes and behaviors or environmental conditions—would continue adding to this list throughout the following two decades. Eating whole grains reduced the risk of type 2 diabetes.[2] It helped people manage obesity.[3] People who ate whole grains had a lower cardiovascular mortality rate and were less likely to get colon cancer.[4]

Researchers were even starting to formulate hypotheses about *why* whole grains protected people from disease. The clearest link was with diabetes prevention: since whole grains are metabolized more slowly than refined grains, they don't come with such a sizable insulin spike. Hence, while the glycemic index of Wonder Bread clocks in at a hefty 73, whole grain bread made with stone-ground flour registers a mere 52.[5] But the glycemic index doesn't explain the links between whole grain consumption and reduced rates of other chronic diseases, like heart disease and cancer. Researchers had a hard time figuring this part out. One hypothesis was that the dietary fiber in whole grains was beneficial for the colon and provided immune protection.[6] Another hypothesis linked health outcomes to the high antioxidant activity of whole grains, pointing out that the antioxidants in these grains were different from those in fruits and vegetables and likely played a unique role in safeguarding the body against disease.[7] Curiously, however, neither hypothesis could account for the full protective effect of a whole grain diet. People who obtained adequate amounts of both fiber and antioxidants from non-grain sources, researchers found, were not as healthy as those who regularly consumed nature's neat package of bran, germ, and endosperm. There was something about whole grain that resisted mechanistic explanations: the whole appeared to be greater than the sum of the parts.[8]

And yet, just as doctors started recommending a diet rich in whole grains, an increasing number of people began reporting that wheat made them sick—bloated, crampy, tired. These "gluten-sensitive" people, as they begin to understand themselves, made up 15–20 percent of the population by some estimates.[9] Gluten-free diets gave them relief but were difficult to follow, given that gluten seemed to be in everything. Gluten-free products exploded onto the market to meet the needs of the rapidly growing ranks of the gluten sensitive, but many of these GF foods were less nutritious than their gluten-containing counterparts. People had to choose between feeling sick and missing out on folates, iron, B vitamins, and fiber.[10]

Researchers started doing studies on gluten, hoping to find some cure for America's suddenly rampant ailment. But very few of them looked at the difference between ancient wheat and modern wheat. In light of the fact that so many people who couldn't digest modern wheat reported better luck with ancient wheat, this seemed like an important question to investigate. By this point, I had already learned the basics of our ancient wheat's nutrient profile: compared with modern wheat, it had higher levels of eight out of nine minerals, 65 percent more amino acids, and 40 percent more protein.[11] Given such major differences in the fundamental composition of this ancient food and its aggressively bred cousins, it was plausible to me that our bodies would metabolize them differently.

I was hearing a lot about how antioxidants were key to the nutritional benefits of certain fruits and vegetables, so I asked Rossana if she knew anybody who could measure the antioxidant capacity of Kamut grain. Earlier tests had shown that this ancient wheat was high in selenium, and it was well-known that selenium was a strong antioxidant, but I wanted to see a definitive study of total antioxidant capacity so I could understand how our grain compared with, say, blueberries. I thought this would be a pretty simple study that someone could do in a test tube.

Rossana also thought the antioxidant question was an interesting one, and she thought researchers would like working with Kamut brand khorasan wheat because the trademark ensured a level of standardization that was difficult to achieve with other ancient wheats, like emmer, spelt, and einkorn. With these other ancient wheats, different strains might have different nutritional properties. In the case of spelt, you might even get varieties that had been crossed with modern wheat— so it could be hard to compare studies and develop a body of literature. Kamut khorasan was legally guaranteed to have a protein content between 12 and 18 percent and a selenium content between 400 and 1,000 parts per billion. It was legally guaranteed to have never been hybridized with modern wheat. We also standardized the growing conditions somewhat by sourcing it all from a specific region and mandating that it be certified organic.

Rossana introduced me to a microbiologist at the University of Bologna and told him about my interest in an antioxidant study. "Sure," he said, "we can do that."

On my next trip to Italy, Rossana took me to visit my new research collaborator, along with his colleague, a nutritional biochemist. I could tell immediately that they made a great team. The microbiologist was affable but a little bit reserved. The nutritional biochemist got right to the point.

"What we would like to propose to you," the nutritional biochemist said, "is a rat study. It's going to cost a lot more money, but it's going to give us better information."

A rat study? That was much more complicated than what I'd envisioned. I thought they could just analyze the grain in a test tube. The sum of money the nutritional biochemist told me was necessary to fund a rat-feeding study was pretty steep. But what she said next made a lot of sense to an organic farmer. With nutrition, as with soil, chemistry gets you only so far.

A test-tube study could only *approximate* the antioxidant activity of our ancient wheat in a living organism, the nutritional biochemist told me. By extracting one compound at a time out of a food—as many whole grain studies were doing at the time—we would be missing the synergies among those compounds, which were likely the source of many of the protective effects. Furthermore, she told me, test-tube studies failed to account for differences in antioxidant solubility and bioavailability within the digestive tract. It was a hopelessly reductive way to look at a complex living system. She didn't say it, but I got the feeling the nutritional biochemist thought this reductive approach was a very American way of doing things.

So we designed a study with five different rat diets. They were all whole grain, and they were all organic. One group of rats was fed bread made with modern wheat. A second group of rats ate bread made with Kamut flour. The third and fourth groups ate modern wheat pasta and Kamut pasta. The microbiologist really wanted to look at the effect of fermentation, so we added a fifth rat diet of sourdough bread made with Kamut flour. I wish we'd spent the extra money to do the modern wheat control on that, but when I think about how far I'd already stretched myself past my initial vision of an antioxidant study in a test tube, I can forgive myself a little bit. And, of course, we had no idea if we'd get any meaningful data at all.

It was a year before we were able to do the study and get the results. Rats introduced a whole new set of complications that wouldn't have come up with a test-tube study. First, there was the matter of experimental design. There are, it turns out, many ways to feed a rat. We decided it was important to give the rats actual human foods rather than just dosing them with grain. But once we'd made that decision, we encountered a second hurdle: there was a committee that needed to verify that the rats would be treated ethically. And even when that committee gave us a green light, some of my friends in the organic community were horrified. They thought this was cruelty to animals. I understood their viewpoint, but I felt nutritional studies using rats were ethically justifiable if it might save human lives or greatly reduce human suffering. I thought about my friend with the environmental sensitivities who said ancient grain made her feel better.

Over the years, I'd heard other equally dramatic testimonials about the health benefits of ancient grain. One lady had called me up, crying, thanking me for growing Kamut grain because she said it was the only grain her daughter could eat. On my first trip to Italy, a fellow came up to me at a food show and said he'd been in very poor health, losing weight, and his doctors had told him there was nothing more they could do to help him. He had thought he was going to die. Ancient grain had made a difference for him too, and he told me that he had been eating Kamut products for several months and was feeling much better. Several years later, I bumped into him again at the food show, and he had made a full recovery, married, and had a child. These were extreme cases and totally unverifiable. But that was exactly why I thought we needed to study the nutritional aspects of ancient wheat—to look at the question scientifically so that doctors and their patients would have reliable information and suffering people could get some answers. Rossana, the Italian naturopath who had connected me with my new research partners, was of the same mind. She signed on to become the director of our research initiative.

When we got the results back from the rat study, our research team ran two different analyses on antioxidant activity, both of which were published in research journals.

The first analysis, published in 2011,[12] looked at the rats that ate bread and measured antioxidant activity in their blood. As I'd hypothesized, we found that the antioxidant capacity of the ancient wheat diet was considerably higher than it was for the modern wheat diet. Rats in the study were given a shot of doxorubicin (known as "dox"), a compound that creates harmful free radicals in the body. Then we analyzed how quickly the rat system was able to eliminate those free radicals, by measuring two markers of oxidative stress in the rats' blood. Rats on the modern wheat diet didn't eliminate very many free radicals, but rats on the ancient wheat eliminated a lot more—a statistically significant difference. They did even better on the sourdough Kamut bread.

As part of the study, the researchers went ahead and looked at the Kamut bread in a test tube too. It had ten times more selenium than modern wheat. But my nutritional biochemist friend was right—the selenium couldn't account for the whole difference between the antioxidant activity levels of the two rat diets. We could have pumped the rats full of selenium and it wouldn't have helped them as much as eating a humble piece of bread.

The second analysis looked at antioxidant activity in the bread-eating rats from another vantage point—enzymes important for reducing oxidative stress in the liver. These findings, published in 2012,[13] were similar: more of the antioxidant liver enzymes were present with the ancient wheat diet than with the modern wheat diet. The researchers also found that some of the antioxidants present in Kamut grain, like ferulic acid, were completely absent from modern wheat. But that second paper also made a curious little side comment.

We'd given our lab rats shots of dox to introduce free radicals so we could measure how fast the rat system could eliminate them. That was antioxidant capacity. But dox has another known side effect, which is inflammation. Researchers who work with dox can see this inflammation under a microscope, particularly in the spleen, lymph nodes, and small intestine.

As we expected, the rats on the modern wheat diet had the telltale signs of inflammation. Their lymphatic follicles—clusters of cells in their spleen and lymph nodes—were visibly enlarged. The lining of their small intestine was flattened, and their villi—the small hairs that help with nutrient absorption in the intestine—were malformed. But the rats on the ancient wheat diet didn't seem to have any of these problems. Could it be that ancient wheat actually protected them from *inflammation* as well as free radicals?

In the preceding decade, a revolution of sorts had occurred in medicine, as studies of a wide range of chronic diseases implicated inflammation as a causal factor in their development. Cancer, cardiovascular disease, diabetes. Autoimmune conditions and nervous system degeneration. Even clinical depression. By the time we were looking at our study rats under a microscope, doctors were beginning to speak of an "inflammation theory of disease," which might in fact unify and advance our understanding of *all* human ailments.[14]

Just as we were puzzling over the surprising results of our study, cardiologist William Davis introduced millions of Americans to this inflammation theory of disease with his best-selling book *Wheat Belly*. Dr. Davis had noticed the same things we had noticed with rats on the modern wheat diet, only in human patients: they had heightened levels of inflammation and they weren't feeling well. Davis put two and two together and warned people against the inflammatory effects of their pretzels, cookies, and bread.

In the opening pages of his book, Dr. Davis placed the blame for modern wheat's health impact squarely on the genetic manipulation of the crop. He even noted that he himself—a strongly wheat-sensitive person—had tried eating ancient wheat and had tolerated it well. But Dr. Davis seemed unaware that ancient wheat was available at a commercial scale and could be a viable alternative. At the end of the book, his recommendation was to simply avoid all wheat, since most wheat products are now made with modern varieties.

I thought Dr. Davis might be interested in our study, so I called him up to tell him what we were seeing in our rats: inflammation with modern wheat, no inflammation with ancient wheat. I told him that the

ancient wheat we had tested—Kamut khorasan—was widely distributed and quite viable for farmers, who were now growing it on tens of
thousands of acres. I was surprised when Dr. Davis wasn't terribly interested. But of course, we hadn't published our data yet, and we hadn't
even designed the study to look at inflammation. It was just an offhand
observation by an attentive researcher.

So I called my research partners in Italy and asked them if they still
had all the rat tissue from the experiment in their freezers. "Oh yes,"
they told me, "everything's here." They were getting ready to publish a
third analysis, this time on the rats that ate pasta.

"Good," I told them. "Look at the tissue from the control rats."

Every good experiment has a control, so we had rats in the experiment that were never given the dox shot. Those rats didn't have any free
radicals added to their system, so they were our baseline to measure how
far above normal our other rats were. Of course, that meant the control
rats also didn't have any inflammation added to their system, at least
not by chemical means. But when we looked at the control rats fed the
modern wheat diet, we found all the telltale signs. Enlarged lymphatic
follicles. Flattened intestinal lining and malformed villi. Dr. Davis was
right! Partly. We had solid evidence that modern wheat caused inflammation. But the control rats on the *ancient* wheat diet didn't have any
of those problems.

So, tacked on to our third paper, the one focused on the rats that
were fed pasta,[15] we added a whole new section on the findings related
to inflammation. We reported all the same results with these rats as we
had with the rats that ate bread: those on the ancient wheat diet had less
oxidative stress, in both the bloodstream and the liver. But then we also
described the striking difference in inflammatory response. The rats on
the modern wheat diet showed all the symptoms: swollen cells in the
spleen, swollen cells in the lymph nodes, malformed small intestines.
The rats on the ancient wheat diet looked normal, even after the shot

of dox, which was known to have an inflammatory affect. The ancient wheat was *counteracting* it.

This was a dramatic finding, with enormous potential implications for human health. But we couldn't just assume that things would be the same for humans as they were for rats. We had to find out.

CHAPTER 14:

Food as Medicine

Forty years prior, when I'd packed my bags for graduate school at UC Davis, I had imagined I'd spend the rest of my life conducting research. Plant research. But medical research? That wasn't something any of my plant science classmates discussed. Health and farming were seen as completely separate fields, so much so that the university saw nothing wrong with establishing its new medical school in Sacramento, twenty miles away from its agricultural faculty. But as I gradually came to understand that how we grow our food affects how it works in the body, I realized that medical research was key to healthy agriculture. So at sixty years of age, after a career of farming and launching rural businesses, I found myself back in the lab.

For our first experimental trial on the effects of an ancient grain diet in humans, we recruited twenty-two healthy volunteers from among the staff of the University of Florence and their family and friends.[1] We took baseline measurements of our subjects for two weeks, then divided them into two groups for a crossover study.

In a crossover study, both experimental groups are given both treatments, in sequence, so you eliminate the potential that some undetected difference in your treatment groups could bias the result. In our case, one group ate pasta, bread, crackers, and biscuits made from whole grain Kamut flour. The other group ate the same foods made from organic, whole grain modern wheat. All of the products were made by the same artisanal manufacturers in Italy. They were pretty tasty, actually. Outside of these products, our subjects were told to continue their normal diet except for wheat—they were only permitted to eat the wheat products that we were providing them.

Each treatment group ate their respective diet for eight weeks. Then they had a washout period for eight weeks, when they all went back to their normal diet. (Over the course of our research, we learned to schedule these washout periods over the holidays, in deference to reality.) Then, for the next eight weeks, the two treatment groups switched diets. That's what made it a crossover study—we looked at each subject on both diets. None of the subjects knew what they were eating, but the researchers did, so it was a single-blind trial.

To measure inflammation in our human subjects, we looked at pro-inflammatory cytokines. Cytokines are signaling molecules that regulate our immune system. In response to immunological stimuli, some cytokines trigger inflammation, which is a good thing if we've just sprained our ankle. When the body sustains an acute injury or is under imminent threat, inflammation can help us protect ourselves and heal. (You may have noticed that physical therapists are no longer telling you to ice your ankle right away if you sprain it—that slows the inflammation, and for the first twenty-four hours or so after an injury, inflammation is actually a good thing.) What we don't want is for inflammation to hang around, keeping our body in a state of stress and high alert. Long-term inflammation saps our energy, disrupts our digestion, and can lead to serious health problems.[2]

Many of the pro-inflammatory cytokines we studied were reduced by 20 to 30 percent on the ancient wheat diet. One of them, tumor necrosis factor, was reduced by 34.6 percent. In just eight weeks! As with the rats, oxidative stress in our human subjects was lower on the ancient wheat diet as well. But that wasn't all. Subjects on the ancient wheat diet also lowered their cholesterol by an average of 4 percent. Low-density lipoprotein (LDL), or "bad" cholesterol, went down by an average of 7.8 percent. The ancient wheat eaters also saw significant decreases in blood glucose. And their levels of iron, potassium, and magnesium went up.

As the medical community began talking more and more about the contribution of inflammation to many types of chronic disease, we realized that the connections between inflammation and disease risk factors were coming into focus right before our eyes. So our research team decided the next logical step was to see if this anti-inflammatory ancient wheat could reduce the risk of things like heart disease and diabetes.

We started our studies of ancient wheat and chronic disease by looking at irritable bowel syndrome, or IBS.[3] One of the challenges of studying human disease is that many people who are sick are taking medication, which introduces a confounding factor to your study. Very large, expensive studies can control for this statistically, as long as the researchers get all the information about what medications their subjects are taking. But our studies were small. So IBS was a good place for us to start, because there aren't any widely used, reliably effective medications for it.

Irritable bowel syndrome was also the most common diagnosis being given to people who claimed they were gluten sensitive, because consumption of wheat and dairy appeared to make IBS worse. It was also thought to be a low-grade inflammatory condition—one group of researchers had even demonstrated a link between IBS diagnoses and cytokine levels.[4] Given what our research team had already learned, the solution of ancient wheat seemed like a plausible fit with the problem of IBS. And with 10 to 20 percent of the population suffering from a condition with no medical cure,[5] enthusiasm for solutions was high.

We recruited patients from the Careggi University Hospital in Florence, all of whom had been diagnosed with IBS. We used the same modern and ancient wheat diets, but this time we used semi–whole wheat flour—a partially refined product—because my research collaborators were afraid that whole wheat might agitate the sensitive intestinal linings of the IBS volunteers and cause them to drop out of the trial.

We followed a similar protocol, but this time we designed a double-blind crossover study. For the first six weeks, one group ate the modern wheat diet and the other group ate the ancient wheat diet. Then they had a washout period, and then they switched diets. It was double-blind because none of the volunteers knew which diet they were eating and the researchers administering it to them didn't know either. All the food in the study was distributed in unmarked packages.

To avoid confounding factors, we again told the study subjects not to eat any wheat during the study (given that they had IBS, they were happy to follow this directive). Then we told them a little bit of a fib. We told them that we were going to give them two types of food and we thought that both diets were going to help them feel better. Now, of course, we didn't really think that the modern wheat was going to help our subjects feel significantly better. But we didn't want to bias our study by leading them to believe that one treatment was effective and one was a dud. Then we'd never know whether the results were just a reflection of the power of persuasion—the placebo effect—or indicated something more fundamental about the difference between ancient and modern wheat. I don't like leading people astray, but all the food was organic, so I thought there might actually be some truth to our statement.

We evaluated our subjects with irritable bowel syndrome in two ways. First, we asked them to keep a weekly diary, recording the severity of each of their symptoms on a hundred-point scale. On the modern wheat diet, our subjects reported almost no difference. When we looked at the graphs of our data, it was just flat lines everywhere. But within six weeks on the ancient wheat diet, they reported significant decreases in all of their symptoms, from fatigue to abdominal pain to bloating to diarrhea. The researchers were astounded—no medicine could produce these kinds of results. Many of the subjects demanded to know what they were eating so they could continue to eat it. (We couldn't tell them during the blinded study, but when they came in for their final physical examination, we sent them home with a letter explaining the study and detailing the foods they had eaten.)

We also did blood tests on our subjects with irritable bowel syndrome, just as we'd done for our first human study with healthy volunteers. The results were nearly identical. Cytokine levels remained relatively constant for subjects on the modern wheat diet. Subjects on the ancient wheat diet, however, saw a 20 to 30 percent reduction in pro-inflammatory cytokines, and one of these cytokines, macrophage inflammatory protein, decreased by 38.9 percent.

The same year we published our irritable bowel syndrome study, the journal *Gastroenterology* published a letter written by two Italian internists titled "Non-Celiac Wheat Sensitivity Is a More Appropriate Label than Non-Celiac Gluten Sensitivity."[6] Many of our IBS subjects had been told they were gluten sensitive, but according to the Italian internists, this probably wasn't the complete picture. Mounting clinical and research evidence suggested that components of wheat other than gluten—lectins, wheat germ agglutinin, or alpha-amylase/trypsin inhibitors—could activate the immune responses involved in so-called gluten sensitivity. All of these components of wheat had been modified through modern breeding, and we were just beginning to understand the effects on the human body. Again, my nutritional biochemist friend was right: you had to look at the whole plant, not just one compound.

Given the promising results we'd seen in healthy volunteers and subjects with irritable bowel syndrome, we decided to see if ancient wheat could help people with heart disease.[7]

Cardiovascular disease causes approximately one-third of deaths globally, and conventional treatment is expensive. Recently, many researchers have shifted their focus from treatment to prevention, finding that food makes a difference. By the time we started conducting our medical trials, studies of the whole grain–rich Mediterranean diet had shown that this pattern of eating could lessen people's chances of dying from heart attack or stroke.[8] In our own study on healthy subjects eating ancient wheat, we had seen reductions in both cholesterol and blood glucose. The next logical question was to put these two data points together and find out whether people who already had serious heart problems could lessen their risks with a specific dietary intervention—substituting ancient wheat for modern wheat.

Most of the people recruited for this study had already had one heart attack. One guy had already had three. Given their high levels of risk, all of these subjects were on statins. Over 80 percent were on beta-blockers, and half took aspirin. Two-thirds were taking somewhere between four and seven different drugs to control their cholesterol and try to prevent another heart attack. Obviously, we weren't going to ask them to stop taking their meds just to eliminate confounding factors in our study.

Unbeknownst to me, however, the researchers conducting the study were managing expectations among themselves as they set up the trial, doubtful that we'd get any meaningful results. We wanted to see if people could lower their cholesterol by eating an ancient grain diet. But the people we were studying were already taking very aggressive drugs to accomplish this same feat. Billions of dollars' worth of research and development had gone into creating these medications. On top of that, our surveys showed that the study participants were adhering fairly well to a Mediterranean diet, even before our intervention. If our subjects were already lowering their cholesterol as much as possible, how could we see any improvement with ancient grains?

We used the same double-blind crossover study protocol we'd used with previous human subjects. We told people they were eating two types of food that would make them feel better, even though our research team wasn't sure we could do anything more for them than they were already doing.

But lo and behold, although our subjects were already reducing their cholesterol with medications, the ancient grain diet brought it down even further: total cholesterol went down by 6.8 percent and LDL dropped by 8.1 percent. Oxidative stress and inflammation went down too, just as we'd seen in the rats and our previous human studies. Additionally, blood glucose, a strong independent predictor of cardiovascular mortality,[9] decreased on the ancient wheat diet by 8 percent.

The other remarkable result we saw in our subjects with cardiovascular risk factors on the ancient wheat diet was a dramatic drop in their insulin levels: 24 percent. This was something we hadn't expected, and it begged an obvious question: could these ancient grains help people with diabetes?

Type 2 diabetes is a chronic condition characterized by excessive glucose levels resulting from insulin resistance or decreased insulin secretion or both. It is estimated that 592 million people will have it by 2035, and it is already an expensive epidemic in industrialized countries. In the United States, one out of every ten health-care dollars is spent on diabetes, which amounts to an annual bill of $245 billion.[10]

Grain presents a dilemma for diabetics. Eating too many carbohydrates can mess with their insulin levels. But low-carb diets can lead to mineral, vitamin, and fiber deficiencies, along with increased cardiovascular risk.[11] A review study, published the same year as our study on heart disease, had found that diabetic patients improved their glycemic control on a Mediterranean diet including whole grains. So we felt confident it was safe to ask patients with diabetes to complete our study protocol.

We recruited patients diagnosed with diabetes from the Careggi University Hospital in Florence and ran our double-blind crossover study.[12] Again, no significant effect was observed on the modern wheat diet. But on the ancient grain diet, subjects' insulin levels went down by 16.3 percent and blood glucose decreased by 9.1 percent. Cholesterol and inflammation went down. Antioxidant capacity went up.

Having seen such dramatic results in patients with multiple forms of metabolic disease—from heart problems to diabetes—we ran one more study, this time with subjects who had been diagnosed with nonalcoholic fatty liver disease. This condition, characterized by an accumulation of fat in the liver, is one of the most serious complications of obesity and impacts an estimated 20–30 percent of the adult population in developed countries. The findings from this study were remarkably similar: a diet of organic, whole grain ancient wheat lowered these patients' cholesterol and inflammation—and also reduced fat in the liver and improved liver function enzymes.[13]

Along the way, we studied some of the mechanisms of ancient wheat's protective effects. We found that it has a more diverse variety of antioxidant compounds than modern wheat, some of which are found *only* in old varieties.[14] We found that it increases levels of health-promoting mutualists of gut microbiota.[15] We also found that environmental conditions on the farm play a fundamental role in determining what nutrients are taken up from the soil and ultimately translated to the wheat kernel.[16] That's one more reason why I've insisted that ancient wheat can't be sold under the name Kamut unless it's raised organically.

More recently, we've been looking into epigenetics. The thinking about genetics used to be that we're all born with a genetic code, an immutable set of instructions for our body. Now, scientists understand that environmental factors turn genes on and off—figuring out *how* and *why* is the work of epigenetics. So we've been looking at the genes that stimulate inflammation in the body. From what we've seen so far, modern wheat turns those genes on. Ancient wheat suppresses them.

What we've been finding in study after study—that differences in wheat *varieties* could have major health implications—poses a monumental challenge to conventional wisdom. Federal dietary guidelines tell us that one strain of wheat is as good as the next. Dr. William Davis basically said the same thing in *Wheat Belly*, although in reverse: one wheat was as bad as the next. Our results departed so dramatically from this way of thinking that initially we had a hard time getting the first papers published. But by the fourth or fifth one, we'd send our paper to an academic journal and the anonymous peer reviews would come back referencing other studies that aligned with our findings.[17] The inquiry into the nutritional differences between ancient and modern wheat was becoming a body of literature. But not quickly enough.

We've now published nearly thirty papers, but our medical trials have been fairly modest in size. Strictly speaking, they are what researchers would call preliminary studies; results found in populations this small should be confirmed with larger groups. We don't have the budget for that (Kamut International has already spent nearly $2 million on this research, modest as it may seem), and if we did, people would probably be skeptical of it. Nutrition science has been badly corrupted by the agricultural-industrial complex, as we've learned from nutritionists like New York University's Dr. Marion Nestle, who traced the sordid history of corporate influence on government dietary guidelines in her book *Food Politics*. Private companies with a horse in the race are not the right people to be funding our nutritional science.

Anyway, our studies have just scratched the surface. I'd like to see an interdisciplinary team from multiple universities apply for a big grant from the National Institutes of Health to compare an ancient wheat diet with a modern wheat diet. They could look at multiple modern grains and multiple ancient grains. Over a longer period of time. With more study subjects.

It shouldn't stop with grain. Now that we know inflammation is implicated in many of our most prevalent chronic diseases, I think we should develop an inflammatory index for our food. Not just ancient wheat versus modern wheat, or heirloom vegetables versus modern vegetables. Organic versus conventional. Whole versus refined. Sourdough versus fast-rising yeast. We should know—at every level, from production through processing—how our food impacts our health, and an inflammatory index seems like a good place to start. Why not put it on a label, as we do with protein and fat and carbohydrates?

For the past three years, I've been working with an Italian researcher to develop a low-cost test of the inflammatory profile of a food, something that could be run for about $100. This researcher has been grinding up cookies made from various flours and exposing them to the same enzymes that live in our stomach, to simulate digestion. Next, he places the predigested cookie grindings in a petri dish along with cell cultures from an actual human gut. Then he monitors what happens—do the cookie grindings create an inflammatory response in the gut cells? To find out, he measures three things. First, he measures cytokines—the same indicators of long-term inflammatory response that we've tracked in our medical trials. Second, he looks at prostaglandins—an indicator of short-term inflammatory response. Finally, he measures the space between the cells to see if some foods lead to greater intestinal permeability—cellular "leaks" in the gut barrier that could allow substances to pass into the bloodstream. The trick with any such mimic of a living system is to eliminate confounding factors to ensure that the results are reliable and reproducible. But I'd much rather we could run these experiments on inflammatory foods in a petri dish so that the public isn't obliged to experiment on their own bodies.

I think there will come a day when we look back at our era the way we now look back at Louis Pasteur and Alexander Fleming and all those people who came up with germ theory. That was revolutionary. We now have much more understanding of infectious disease, and in areas of the world with sufficient resources, it is no longer a major cause of death. This is not just because doctors know how to *treat* infectious disease but also because non–medical professionals and the general public know how to *prevent* it. In early nineteenth-century London, thousands of people died from cholera because the city was disposing of human waste in the same river that served as a major supply of drinking water.[18] Our civil engineers know better than that now.

Now we are at the very beginning of another revolution in the understanding of disease. This will be a more subtle revolution, but a critically important one, because it will transform our understanding of how our bodies function, how our food functions, and how they affect each other. It will also be a more contested revolution.

When I was a young boy, all of society celebrated Jonas Salk's vaccination for polio. Americans of all backgrounds understood this as a victory for public health. But when pioneering researchers started asking questions about the links between food and health, there were some conspicuous non-celebrators. The agricultural-industrial complex and the big pharmaceutical companies don't want these questions asked. It's a direct threat to their business model and to their fiduciary responsibility to make as much money as possible. You know what they would do with polio today? Focus all their money on building a better iron lung. That would benefit the iron lung manufacturers, and because they would have the biggest, most well-funded lobby, that's where the money would go.

Sooner or later, though, we are going to have to get serious about diet-related disease. Today, nearly one in three people on the planet suffers from a disease related to what they do (or do not) eat. Many of these people are children. In 2016, 155 million of the world's children under the age of five were undernourished, while 41 million were overweight or obese. These diet-related conditions account for nearly half of the global child mortality rate.[19] In the United States alone, unhealthy diets contribute to 678,000 deaths each year. In the past three decades, US obesity rates have doubled in adults, tripled in children, and quadrupled in teenagers. Currently, over two-thirds of American adults are either overweight or obese.[20]

No country can afford to have a significant percentage of its population chronically ill. I don't care what kind of a health-care system we have; we can't afford that. We're doing the same thing with the American population that my chemical farming neighbors are doing to their soil: spending more and more money in a losing battle to treat symptoms when we ought to be focused on addressing the root cause of the problem—why are so many people sick?

Each year, obesity care costs Americans $147 billion. Diabetes accounts for another $116 billion. It's hard to parse the additional costs for diet-related cardiovascular disease and cancer, but these would add additional hundreds of billions to the tab.[21] And these numbers don't begin to address the economic costs of lost work hours or the human costs of pain and suffering. "Cheap" food ruins lives.

And yet, we're still growing this stuff, millions of acres of commodity corn and wheat for high-fructose corn syrup and Wonder Bread. We're still breeding principally for yield rather than asking how all these genetic modifications to our foods are impacting their contribution to our health and our ability to digest them. I think farmers would be up in arms about this if they thought about it, but the commodity mindset distracts farmers from the fact that what they are growing is not just a widget but someone's dinner. If you wanted to make a very hard bingo game, you could send people to a mainstream farm convention and give them a point every time they heard the word "food." It's all commodities, commodities, commodities. Very few farmers eat their own wheat, so that widens the disconnect between agriculture and food, agriculture and health.

I wish more of my fellow plant biochemists were working to bridge this gap, because they could do a lot to help us understand how plants mediate the relationship between soil and the human digestive tract. But increasingly, I collaborate with people from all sorts of disciplines, from paleobotanists to cell biologists. The way I see it, these are just different windows into the same house.

CHAPTER 15:

One Great Subject

The British soil scientist Sir Albert Howard once wrote that the health of soil, the health of plants, the health of animals, and the health of people should all be studied as one great subject. It wasn't Howard's idea. He learned it from peasant farmers in India who taught him how to compost when he was stationed there in 1905 to "improve" the agriculture of this recently established British colony. To his credit, Sir Albert was a smart man and a good listener. Although he was sent to the Indian subcontinent to convert peasant farmers to modern Western agricultural methods, he ended up learning more from his purported students than he felt he had to teach them. The knowledge Sir Albert Howard brought back from his travels in India became the cornerstone of the organic farming movement that developed in both England and the United States in the mid-twentieth century.

In the context of the rapid industrialization of the Western world, this organic movement was understood as alternative, unorthodox. Okay, weird. But this link between diet and farming, land health and human health, is written into just about every wisdom tradition on the face of the planet. Native Hawaiians refer to land as 'āina, "that which feeds," and the term also connotes a family bond between humans, plants, and the earth.[1] The Bible teaches that people were created from soil and placed in a garden to till and tend it.[2] In ancient Greece, the physician Hippocrates famously counseled, "Let food be thy medicine and medicine be thy food." The only culture that seems to be lacking such a teaching is our own. But that might be changing.

When I was just getting my start as an entrepreneur, in the 1980s, the word "sustainability" began to enter common parlance. The United Nations published the Brundtland Report on sustainable development in 1987, and the phrase "triple bottom line" was coined in 1994 by entrepreneur John Elkington.[3] Taking a triple bottom line approach to one's business meant accounting for three types of value added (or subtracted) by business operations: not just profit but also value to people and planet. This was a revolutionary concept for businesses that had previously externalized costs like environmental damage and health problems for workers exposed to toxins. But even sustainability-oriented businesses still tended to see these three bottom lines as separate goals, and given their overriding obligations to their shareholders, profit frequently trumped people and planet.

In my early days running the grain business, this was my perspective too. My goal in starting the business had been to add economic value to my farm so that it could support two families. Pretty quickly, that goal expanded to include adding economic value to my neighbors' crops and creating jobs in our rural community. I started to see the "people" part of the triple bottom line at that point, and once I started sourcing organic wheat, my customers told me why they thought that was better for the planet. But it wasn't until I started converting my own farm to organic that I began to see that these forms of value were tightly linked: investing in a healthy soil added economic and environmental value at the same time. The triple bottom line wasn't a matter of managing three separate ledgers—this was about finding the synergies among all these benefits, which was where the real value was. Getting involved in medical studies really brought home for me how *people* fit into the equation, as I realized that the human body was integrating a great deal of information about the entire life story of our food—how it was processed, how it was grown, and even how the genetics of its ancestors had been modified over time by farmers or scientists. The subjects of those medical studies showed me just how closely the health of our bodies is connected to the health of our surroundings: our planet, our farms, and our communities.

Three decades after finishing my PhD and leaving academia, I was more excited than ever about pursuing research. Not in the manner in which I'd been trained, dissecting plants and analyzing them at the biochemical level, but in the manner Sir Albert Howard had suggested: taking the health of people, plants, animals, and soils as one great subject. Not many researchers were following Howard's advice, but one who was got my attention.

When the Montana Organic Association convened its annual meeting in 2006, in Missoula, we invited a guest speaker from Washington State University: a six-foot-five wheat breeder named Stephen Jones.

Steve's academic background was not too dissimilar from mine: he had gone to UC Davis for his PhD and been steeped in the principles and practices of agribusiness. He had even landed a plum faculty job at a leading agricultural university for wheat, Washington State. When Steve released a variety, it had the potential to be planted on hundreds of thousands of acres.

But Steve never liked the idea of a single wheat variety being planted on hundreds of thousands of acres. He thought monoculture was artificial, and it bothered him to see commodity wheat varieties getting less and less nutritious and flavorful. So, in addition to his formal responsibilities, he started breeding more distinctive varieties for organic farmers, who had been left out to dry by conventional breeding programs. Conventional varieties were optimized to respond to generous applications of synthetic fertilizer—which meant they did not shine under organic management.[4] Steve was one of the first wheat breeders developing varieties specifically for high performance in organic systems, so we were all eager to hear what he had to say. It was one of the best presentations we'd ever had.

Meanwhile, Steve's department back at Washington State had been pursuing another direction for the future of wheat: biotech. Monsanto, eager to commercialize a genetically modified wheat, was angling for partnerships with university researchers who could develop a Roundup Ready wheat, recommend it to farmers, and share in the royalties. Steve tried to quietly avoid such overtures, believing that his duty as a public plant breeder was to serve the public interest and that GMO wheat didn't fit the bill. But eventually he was called into a series of meetings with officials from the Washington Grain Commission, university administrators, and Monsanto reps. They asked him to breed the Roundup Ready wheat. Steve said no.[5]

Steve didn't lose his job, but things got pretty unpleasant for him. Eventually, he decided to leave his faculty position on campus and transfer to the university's Mount Vernon Research and Extension Center in the Skagit Valley, an area known mostly for its annual tulip festival. He figured he was done with wheat. But on the drive to his new job, Steve noticed small farmers planting the staple grain—as a rotation crop to build their soil for more flowers and vegetables. He asked the farmers if they would be interested in working with distinctive varieties that could fetch a premium in Seattle's artisanal bakeries.[6]

In 2011, Steve carved out a little space at Mount Vernon that he called the Bread Lab. He had already been crossing varieties of wheat with interesting characteristics—high micronutrient content, striking colors, adaptability to Western Washington soils—and inviting farmers to try them out and give him feedback.[7] But the Bread Lab didn't just invite farmers. The new lab became a meeting ground for the entire wheat supply chain, from millers to bakers to maltsters.[8] Steve got them equipment, so they could come in and play with his thousands of different varieties. A farinograph to measure the strength of the dough. An alveograph to measure elasticity.[9] And a steam-injected hearth oven that even the choosiest bakers and chefs would drool over.[10] I began sending Steve wheat varieties that I was trialing in my experimental plots so he could test their suitability for bread.

As I had learned from my work with colleagues in Italy, people's preference for foods that taste and smell good isn't just a matter of pleasure. It's also a matter of evolution: our senses have evolved to guide us toward meals that are nutritious and steer us clear of fare that might be toxic. Aggressive marketing and addictive doses of sugar, salt, and trans fat have manipulated our sensory intelligence, but good, real food can help us redevelop it. Such was the case with Steve's breads. Working with nutritionists, the Bread Lab found high levels of polyphenols and other secondary plant metabolites in the organic grain being used in many of the recipes, which meant antioxidant and anti-inflammatory benefits. Meanwhile, the bakers found that these same micronutrients produced distinctive flavors and tantalizing aromas, for which their customers developed a hankering.

It wasn't long before the Bread Lab started turning out mouthwatering new creations: loaves that had "chocolaty overtones and a hint of spice." Loaves that were off the charts in iron content. Loaves that were purple.[11] Steve wanted people to see—and taste—the tremendous potential of wheat that had been left behind in the single-minded pursuit of high-yielding varieties for industrial white bread. Within a few years, Chipotle Mexican Grill came calling for consultation on its tortillas.[12] Bill Gates dropped by too. In 2017, the coterie of mad bread scientists moved into a new 12,000-square-foot facility at the Port of Skagit, complete with a new baking school.[13] But the best part was the conversations: farmers talking protein content with nutritionists and bakers talking with biologists about reviving people's ability to use their sense of taste as a guide to healthy food. Here in the Skagit Valley, Steve was building a literal nose for value right into the food culture.

As a free-range researcher, I've tried to do what I can to advance this sort of integrated understanding of food and agriculture, with the nutrition studies we've funded in Italy and the test plots on my own farm. In addition to the studies I've done with dryland vegetables and fruit trees, I've experimented with a number of other crops that I think could boost food security, environmental stewardship, and human health at the same time.

One of the most remarkable crops I've worked with in my test plots is Painted Mountain Corn, a brightly colored, antioxidant-rich grain corn that has been the life's work of self-taught Montana plant breeder Dave Christensen. Painted Mountain Corn is open-pollinated, meaning the seeds can be saved and replanted by farmers. Unlike the hybrid and GMO varieties most commonly raised by commercial American corn farmers, Painted Mountain Corn is a kind of modern landrace, bred to be genetically diverse for resilience in all manner of challenging growing conditions without the use of chemical fertilizer, pesticides, or irrigation. Rather than trying to earn a Guinness World Record for corn yields under perfect conditions (as it appears some of our midwestern universities are endeavoring to do), Dave has bred this corn to yield adequately to meet human needs under the kinds of conditions most food-insecure people face: sparse rainfall, nutrient-poor soils, and in some cases wind and cold. Among the places Dave has been asked to introduce this corn is North Korea, where it is grown in the cold northern provinces.

I've also experimented with intercropping—planting two crops in the same field at the same time. In my case, I'm interested in whether I can grow my nitrogen fertility right along with my crop by undersowing peas in my barley and Kamut fields. The peas are a completely different shape from the grains, so it's fairly easy to separate them after harvest with a simple cleaning machine. Figuring out the proper timing of planting and harvesting is tricky, though, and the biggest challenge is ensuring adequate moisture. But if we could develop a reasonably reliable protocol for this kind of intercropping, it might help farmers who worry that they can't afford to plant soil-building crops because they're counting on the income from planting cash crops on all their fields, every year. A Kamut-pea intercrop would essentially allow them to cash crop and cover crop at the same time, ensuring that the soil would have adequate nitrogen and thus the grain would have adequate protein.

I'm still experimenting with my cover crop rotation as well, along with the ever-present challenge of organic weed management. I've also done a trial of my dryland squash varieties to see which ones best retain their quality and nutritional value in storage. In addition, I've had a number of interns initiate their own research projects at the farm—including Jacob Cowgill, whose experiments here with heritage animals and grains were the germ of the operation that he and his wife, Courtney, now run in Power, Montana: Prairie Heritage Farm. And the full-time field person we've hired to work with Kamut growers has a research mission too: not just to solve today's problems but also to use the data set compiled by our grower network to try to solve tomorrow's.

In the coming year or two, all these research activities on my farm will be organized into a 600-acre organic research center affiliated with the Rodale Institute in Pennsylvania. Since my first subscription to Rodale's *Organic Gardening* magazine, I've had great respect for the Rodale Institute's research. The institute's Farming Systems Trial has been going for

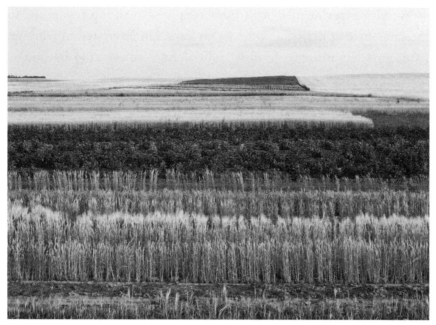

RESEARCH PLOTS IN EARLY SUMMER, WITH DRYLAND POTATOES SANDWICHED
BETWEEN GRAIN TRIALS. THE LAST TWO PLOTS, AT THE BACK OF THE PHOTO,
ARE PLANTED TO PAINTED MOUNTAIN CORN AND INDUSTRIAL HEMP.
(Photo by Hilary Page)

nearly forty years now, since 1981, and it has provided some of the most
definitive information available on the long-term impacts of organic
farming on soil health. Most agricultural trials are carried out for only
two or three years, which doesn't tell you much about gradual processes
like building up soil organic matter. Rodale's study demonstrates what
can be accomplished over a lifetime of farming.

And yet, as I learned when I was converting my own farm to organic,
although the principles are universal, the practices are place specific.
Rodale's farm is very well suited to Kutztown, Pennsylvania. But we
can't copy everything they do and make it work in chilly, semi-arid Big
Sandy, Montana. So I thought we should establish an organic research
center here.

When I contacted friends at Rodale about my idea to launch a research center, they were delighted. It turns out they had already been working on a similar plan of their own: a network of regional centers that could all contribute to comparative studies on major research questions but also study problems specific to their regions. We decided part of my farm could be one of them.

We envision a staff of three: A full-time research director who will manage and set up the experiments. A full-time technical field person who will help carry out the experiments (including the ones I've started) and gather data. Plus a third person, an extensionist, to answer questions from farmers, organize field days in the summer, and offer workshops in the winter. I'll donate the land and seed the research center's budget with some Kamut International stock, and we're working out an arrangement for the center to use my farm machinery in exchange for crop shares so they don't have to take on that big capital expense up front. The center will serve the northern Great Plains, including the western Dakotas and Southern Alberta and Saskatchewan, as well as parts of the dry plains of Wyoming, Colorado, and Nebraska. We hope we can make some modest progress on Sir Albert Howard's "one great subject."

An increasingly important topic for our research center—and others—will be the great challenge facing our children and grandchildren: climate change. When I was a kid, I planted watermelons every year, even though they seldom grew bigger than a softball. They never got ripe. Even the ones that got a little pink didn't taste that great. A few years ago, I bought a few watermelon plants just for fun. I ended up with a thirty-five-pound watermelon. It was delicious. Perfectly ripe.

When I was growing up, we'd have a severe hailstorm once every fifteen years or so. In the past five years, we've had four years with significant hail.

Three years ago, we had a record wet year. The next year was a record dry year and a record fire season, with extreme heat arriving earlier in the spring and lingering longer into the fall.

Between the rain and the drought and the hail, it's becoming riskier and riskier for us to grow spring crops. Even in an average year these days, it gets too dry too quick and too hot too quick. So one of my research projects has been to see if I can find spring crops with enough winter hardiness that we could plant in the fall and harvest early the next season, as we do with our winter wheat.

But adapting to climate change isn't just about selecting more cold-tolerant or drought-tolerant varieties. It's definitely not just about buying more crop insurance, which is too often used to prop up failing farm systems at taxpayers' expense. We need to make more fundamental changes to the way we farm, and one of the most critical is a dramatic increase in biodiversity. I've learned my lesson about diversity the hard way over the years, and a few seasons ago I got a sobering reminder.

It was not the first hailstorm I'd seen ravage our farm. On the north central Montana prairie, every farmer knows the "big white combine" is coming sooner or later. But this hailstorm was unlike any I'd ever seen. The stones were smaller, but the torrent lasted longer. This posed a completely novel challenge to my crops.

When the hailstorm blew through, my feed barley was nearly ripe. The tiny hailstones peeled all the kernels off the barley, so only the stems were left standing. It was a 100 percent loss.

The winter wheat was not quite ready to be harvested, so it was not so easily shelled out. But that was pretty beat up too—about a 60 percent loss.

Fortunately, the Kamut plants weren't as far along. The kernels weren't readily stripped from the plant because they weren't as ripe and were still held more tightly in the head. We had only a 20 or 25 percent loss on that.

The safflower had just started blooming. No seeds had developed yet, so there was almost no damage to those plants. They were bruised a little, but everything continued to develop and seemed fine.

The alfalfa hay had already been cut and baled. There was no loss there because it had already been harvested.

Not a great season, certainly, but not a disaster either. Thanks to the diversity of my crops and their life cycles, my farm was able to weather the storm, while some of my neighbors lost their entire crop. I didn't reach any new milestones for yield, but I got by. It's not the kind of year I'm used to thinking of as a success, because success in American farming during my lifetime has been defined by maximizing volume in the good years. But those good years have always been few and far between in variable weather conditions like ours, and they're getting scarcer. So in the era of climate change, I think we need to rethink our definition of an agricultural success story. It's not about being the biggest and the best. It's about resilience.

CHAPTER 16:

Rejecting the Status Quo

If there's all this value just waiting to be added to our food system, why aren't more farmers and eaters trying to realize it? Organic, perhaps the best-known segment of the value-added food sector, has grown substantially since I converted my farm, to the point where 82 percent of US households purchase at least some organic food.[1] Montana, I'm proud to say, is above the national average, with 85 percent of households including organic items in their grocery cart.[2] But overall, organics still account for just 5.3 percent of US food sales[3] and less than 1 percent of American cropland.[4] Why haven't more of us converted?

This question used to puzzle me, because organic seemed like such a win-win-win proposition: tastier and more nutritious for eaters, more economical for farmers, and healthier for farmland and the surrounding environment. As a scientist, I also thought these systems would be much more interesting for researchers to study (compared with eking out tiny little marginal increases in the yields of a few staple crops), so I was puzzled by the fact that so few of them did.[5]

It wasn't until I began promoting organic agriculture at mainstream farm conventions that I started to realize there was one big loser in the transition to organics: agribusiness. Organic farmers don't need most of the products sold by agribusiness. Nor do we reliably sell our food into their lucrative industrial processing facilities and retail outlets, where they can take their cut. When farmers and artisans and eaters capture more of the value in our food system, that means less of it is left for these input dealers and large, consolidated processors. What I eventually came to understand is that one of the main reasons organic food has yet to go mainstream is that it poses an existential threat to a major multinational industry, and that industry is fighting tooth and nail to protect its fundamentally flawed business model.

The rhetorical strategy currently being employed by agribusiness is common to most outmoded industries: first, they argue that the status quo is just fine. When that argument begins to wear out, they try to convince you that change is dangerous. At the risk of getting too polemical, I want to squarely address both of those claims.

"The Status Quo Is Just Fine"

I'll say this bluntly: Monsanto has lied to us. They've told us their chemicals are safe, and they're not.

Pesticide exposure has been linked to increased incidence of Alzheimer's disease, cancer, birth defects, asthma, Parkinson's disease, sterility, and learning and developmental disorders.[6] I've seen this happen right before my eyes in Big Sandy.

Glyphosate—marketed by Monsanto as Roundup—was billed as a safer alternative to earlier herbicides known to cause health problems. Worldwide use has skyrocketed, such that by 2010, sales of glyphosate exceeded the value of all other herbicides combined.[7] But evidence of Roundup-related health concerns has been mounting,[8] and a recent meta-analysis by the International Agency for Research on Cancer concluded that glyphosate is a "probable carcinogen."[9] Limiting exposure is nearly impossible. A 2011 test of soybean samples by the US Department of Agriculture found glyphosate residue on over 90 percent of them.[10] Recently released internal documents from the US Food and Drug Administration reveal glyphosate residues in crackers, granola, and cornmeal.[11] On my own organic farm, our tests show that traces of the chemical are in our rainwater.

Chemical companies tell us we can trust their products because they have to go through rigorous testing to enter the market. But they do much of this testing themselves, one chemical at a time, for short periods of time. Only chemicals listed as active ingredients are tested—not the compounds they break down into, nor the solvents, adjuvants, and surfactants used in the product formulations that are sold to farmers and applied on crops. We have very few independent studies to tell us what the long-term impact of low exposure might be, particularly under real-life conditions, in which we may experience synergistic effects of multiple chemicals. The studies that have attempted to address these real-life pesticide exposures report very concerning levels of endocrine disruption linked to cancers of the reproductive tissues: breast, prostate, testicles. Children are at the most risk: pesticide exposure in early childhood and in utero can disrupt brain development, leading to lifelong health problems.[12]

Pesticides also harm other organisms we humans depend on, like pollinators. Approximately one-third of food production depends on animal pollinators, such as bees, and three-quarters of all fruits and vegetables increase their production when visited by these keystone organisms.[13] Lately, however, pollinators have experienced steep global population declines. Honeybee colony losses have climbed to as high as 30 percent in the United States in recent years,[14] while the relative abundance of certain bumblebee species has declined by 96 percent.[15] In Europe, nearly one-quarter of bumblebee species face extinction.[16] Pesticides have hit these pollinators with a one-two punch: overuse of herbicides eliminates their habitat,[17] while overuse of neonicotinoid insecticides (frequently used as a coating on conventional seeds) kills them directly.[18]

Maddeningly, the more chemicals we use, the less effective they are. There are now 210 species of herbicide-resistant weeds, many of them resistant to glyphosate.[19] My neighbors are now turning to cocktails of herbicides and going back to even more toxic chemicals like paraquat, dicamba, and 2,4-D. This treadmill of increasing chemical use and increasing resistance exacerbates everything: the health problems, the environmental problems, and the increasing cost to farmers, who already operate on razor-thin margins.

Meanwhile, decades of chemical fertilizer application are acidifying farm soils,[20] and fertilizer runoff has contaminated not only rural drinking water supplies but also urban communities downstream and even ocean ecosystems at the mouths of rivers.[21] The vast fertilizer runoff into the Mississippi River Watershed has fueled a dead zone the size of New Jersey in the Gulf of Mexico, which is now impacting the health of that ecosystem as well as the viability of thousands of small fishing operations.[22]

What's more, fertilizers pollute our environment long before we use them. That huge swath of global greenhouse gas emissions attributed to the food system—as high as one-third of total emissions, by some estimates?[23] Those emissions are due in no small part to energy-intensive fertilizer manufacture,[24] along with industrial methods of raising livestock in confinement. Organic systems not only eliminate these synthetic fertilizers but actually have considerable potential to sequester carbon, thereby transforming agriculture from a climate change problem to a climate change solution.[25]

"Change Is Dangerous"

Once you start to research the impact of chemical agriculture, it's hard to sustain the belief that the status quo is fine. That's when agribusiness tries to convince you that its products are a necessary evil and that abandoning them could lead to mass starvation.

This is the message I get when I go to conventional ag meetings or pick up mainstream ag publications: we need chemical agriculture to feed the world. This statement is based on two faulty assumptions, both of which are actively promulgated by the agrichemical-industrial complex. The first assumption is that achieving global food security is primarily a matter of increasing the yield potential of grain monocultures under ideal conditions. The second assumption is that chemical agriculture is the only way to do it.

Let's start with the first assumption and consider the current state of global food security. Today, at the global scale, agriculture produces a food surplus. Yet 2 billion people are chronically hungry or malnourished.[26] It simply cannot be the case that high yields lead to food security, because we've overshot the yield mark and still the world is not fed.

Moreover, crop yields don't correlate particularly well with food security. Studies of child undernutrition—a key indicator of food insecurity—point toward gender equity and women's education as more important variables in explaining disparities among countries.[27]

The problem, it turns out, isn't *lack* of food. The problem is that many people cannot afford it, including a significant share of the world's farmers.[28] When you sell raw materials low and purchase finished products high, you run out of money to put food on your own table, even if you're the one growing the ingredients. This is why yield increases failed to solve the twentieth century's hunger crisis: the export logic of industrial agriculture has often deepened poverty, which tends to be the root cause of hunger.

But the twenty-first century's hunger crisis, some researchers argue, will be different. Given this century's projected population growth and climate impacts on agriculture, we may actually experience a *global* food shortage. Now more than ever, we need higher-yielding crops, but I'm not so sure. How much more grain can we get out of a wheat plant, after pushing its genetics to the brink for over fifty years? At this point, if we truly want to increase global food availability, I think we should ease up on striving for incremental yield gains in crop breeding and put more of our focus on two problems with far more room for improvement: food waste and dietary composition.

In developed countries like the United States, we waste 30 to 50 percent of our food, mostly in supermarkets, restaurants, and homes. In developing countries, rates of food waste can be as high as 35 percent—typically because farmers lack adequate storage and transportation to get food to market without spoiling.[29] These are problems we could solve.

Dietary shift offers another golden opportunity to improve global food security. Over the past century, Americans have developed a near obsession with grain-fed meat. We like it because it's marbled, a nice way of saying "fatty." But cramming all this grain into our livestock is not good for our cattle, which evolved to eat grass. It's not good for us, either—diets heavy in fatty meat have been linked to heart disease, stroke, type 2 diabetes, obesity, and certain cancers. What's more, it's a terrific waste. More than half the protein produced on croplands comes from feed crops, but only 26 percent of it ends up in human diets, due to the inefficiency of running nutrients through an animal. (The math is even worse for calories: more than one-third of the calories produced on cropland come from feed crops, but only 4 percent of them end up in human diets.)[30]

Rather than raising our cattle on grain that could be used to feed people, it would be much more sensible to raise them on grass. It's what they evolved to eat, after all, and we have millions of acres of rangeland in the western United States that are unsuitable for growing crops but great for pasturing livestock. Were we to ditch our fatty meat in favor of grass-fed and cut global meat consumption in half, we could feed an additional 2 billion people on the same resource base we have now.[31] I used to think ditching grain-fed meat was a sensible sacrifice to make—until I traveled to Argentina, a country where grass-fed beef is the norm. Let me assure you, eating properly prepared grass-fed beef is no sacrifice.

As for the second assumption—that chemical agriculture is necessary to produce adequate yields—its credibility is greatly diminished once you've pulled the curtain back on the role of yields in global food security. But holding aside the spuriousness of the yield-hunger link for the moment, it's worth addressing the matter of just how much food can be grown in organic systems—because there's good evidence to suggest that the yield advantages of chemical agriculture have been overstated.

A large 2007 meta-analysis—a statistical summary of numerous research findings on a single topic—found that organic yields in developed countries were about 8 percent lower than conventional yields.[32] A more recent meta-analysis found the same 8 percent "yield gap" when comparing organic farming systems with complex crop rotations to chemical agriculture.[33] As one researcher pointed out, if this yield gap holds across all global agriculture, reducing food waste by half would do more to boost global food security than chemical agriculture, and with much better outcomes for human health and the planet.[34]

However, it's not clear that even this 8 percent yield gap exists everywhere. The 2007 meta-analysis found that in developing countries (where most of the world's people live), organic farms outperformed low-input conventional farms by up to 80 percent.[35] And the Rodale Institute's side-by-side trials of conventional and organic farming—among the few truly long-term studies we have on the question—have found equivalent yields across chemical and organic plots, in both corn-soy systems and wheat systems.

An important parameter to pay attention to in such studies is whether they are designed to measure the total amount of food produced in a given area or just yields of one crop. Organic farmers often take advantage of synergies among multiple crops and plant them together, thereby increasing the total productivity of the land beyond what is possible with chemical monocultures.[36] One analysis predicted that an organic farming strategy focused on careful crop rotation and polycultures could double African food production in just three to ten years.[37]

Where organics really win out is in the long game. By returning nutrients and organic matter to the soil, organic farmers can sustain yields for thousands of years.[38] Chemical farming, which is not even a century old, is already foundering. A recent analysis of global staple crops found that 24 to 39 percent of regions growing corn, soy, rice, or wheat saw their yields stagnate or collapse between 1961 and 2008.[39] The factors involved are numerous—ranging from depletion of irrigation water to buildup of pests and diseases to lack of capital required to continuously purchase the inputs necessary for achieving high yields with modern varieties. But suffice it to say, industrial agriculture is not the silver bullet it has been made out to be. And as chemical agriculture continues to undermine the resources it relies on—from a stable climate to freshwater reserves to a reliable population of pollinators—the ground is literally shifting under its feet. Over 20 percent of land on Earth is currently classified as degraded, due in no small part to the abuses of industrial agriculture.[40]

Many of the world's farmers live in regions already feeling the stresses of climate change. I know I do. These pressures will almost certainly get worse before they get better, even under best-case scenarios of global action to limit greenhouse gas emissions. We're going to have more droughts, more storms, more new insect pests, all of which will be difficult to predict. Chemical monocultures will fail spectacularly under such conditions, as we're already seeing with Cavendish bananas—the single cultivar that accounts for nearly all of the multibillion-dollar banana export business and is now being devastated by a deadly fungus.[41] In our warming world, organic farming is our best shot for resilience, because diverse crop rotations spread risk and organically managed soils are better at storing water and reducing runoff and erosion.[42] A recent study at the Rodale Institute found that organic corn yields were 31 percent higher than conventional in years of drought. The researchers at Rodale also trialed a genetically modified corn that had been engineered for drought tolerance. The GMO variety did outperform conventional yields in years of drought—but by only 6.7 to 13.3 percent.

Of course, we don't just want agriculture to *feed* the world; we want it to *nourish* the world. Here again, industrial agriculture is failing, as modern varieties show lower levels of both macronutrients and micronutrients.[43] The problem is made worse by the way in which these extractive agricultural systems degrade soils: even if the crops were bred to scavenge more nutrients, they wouldn't find many where they're growing. Conversely, diverse agricultural production has been linked to dietary diversity and better nutrition,[44] and organic crops demonstrate substantially higher levels of antioxidants.[45]

A False Solution

The agricultural-industrial complex has a third card in hand, which is the argument that they recognize all these problems and have devised a revolutionary solution: genetically engineered crops. In describing these biotech products, they use many of the same words organic farmers have used to describe their systems: "sustainable," "ecological," "green."

Don't be fooled.

These are chemical companies, attempting to diversify their portfolios and ensure a market for their core products at the same time. Although biotechnology advocates like to talk about humanitarian-sounding applications for their products, the reality is that the vast majority of biotech crops actually in production are engineered for resistance to one of Monsanto's herbicides: glyphosate (marketed as Roundup) or dicamba.[46] Despite Monsanto's claim that Roundup Ready crops would decrease herbicide use,[47] the opposite has happened. In the twenty years since these genetically engineered crops were introduced, overall herbicide use in the United States has risen by 21 percent,[48] and glyphosate use has more than doubled.[49] Now its effectiveness is wearing off as weeds adapt to resist it, so farmers have to go back to Monsanto and buy more herbicide, like dicamba. I don't think Monsanto's executives are disappointed.

Locking in a chemically intensive system of agriculture is profitable. Really profitable. But somebody has to pay for all those profits, and as the agrichemical-industrial complex pushes to take its model global, I wonder who is going to foot the bill. Consider that farmers in the United States, one of the richest nations in the world, have had to rely on massive government subsidies to cover the costs of high-input agriculture. Even still, large numbers of them have gone out of business or sunk into deep debt. Does the rest of the world really want to follow that example?

The multinational corporations that have been hoarding all the profits from our food system have used their large coffers to exercise tremendous influence over policy makers and researchers. At the same time, they've tried to win over public opinion with information campaigns designed to convince us that their products are safe, that abandoning them is dangerous, and that we need their expensive proprietary biotech to feed the world. I don't buy it. The value in our food system belongs to all of us. It's time to take it back.

CHAPTER 17:

Conclusion: A New Generation of Growers and Eaters

Imagine I told you there was a product that could dramatically reduce the incidence of four of the top seven causes of death in the United States,[1] lift thousands of Americans out of poverty, and fight climate change—all while slowing the growth of marine dead zones and reversing pollinator decline.

If this were an app, venture capitalists would be falling all over themselves to fund it. If it were a new gadget, it would be making headlines and winning awards. But the common solution that an increasing number of people are now proposing as a response to these problems is not a new app. It's not a new gadget. Rather, it's about revaluing something we've come to take for granted: our food.

A regenerative organic food and agriculture system is the only way out of the chronic disease problems plaguing this country. Many are calling it the most promising means of dealing with climate change. And given that seven of the ten lowest-paying jobs in our economy are in this sector,[2] we're not going to solve poverty without reforming food. So why aren't we making bolder moves in this direction?

We Americans like to think of ourselves as an independent, self-sufficient lot. At the core of our national story is the idea that only a people capable of meeting its own needs can fashion a truly free society. Ever since the women of the American Revolution wove their own homespun goods to avoid purchasing imports from the British, do-it-yourself has been baked into our democracy.

Once the American colonists established political independence from the oligarchies of Europe, they were keen to establish economic independence as well and prevent the rise of an equally oligarchical society in the New World. Thus, the founders of this country envisioned it as a nation of small farms: self-determining households that could produce most of their own goods and sell the surplus to pay for equipment or luxuries. It's true that the ideal hasn't always stood up to reality. When Thomas Jefferson wrote about agrarian democracy, he did so from a plantation run on slave labor. My own farm lies near tribal land, where Native Americans still suffer the consequences of a long history of displacement and violence. These shameful legacies can't be swept under the rug when we wax poetic about America's past. Yet I am heartened when I think about one simple statistic: in 1820, 72 percent of Americans listed their primary job as a "farming occupation."[3] The value of what they produced was self-evident: it was directly useful to the household that made it.

Over the following century and a half, the American economy diversified into other goods besides food and fiber. But if we weren't exclusively a nation of small farmers, we nonetheless remained a nation of producers. With much of what Americans made and used circulating in the domestic economy, people still had a notion of quality that was connected to their own experience creating something from scratch. Homesteaders were in the minority by the early twentieth century, but even urban American families had the capacity to produce much of what they needed, from bread to clothing to quilts. These skills proved vital when America sank into a deep depression in the 1930s and families had to get by with little cash. Such skills proved equally important in the following decade when the United States went to war and the country's manufacturing infrastructure was needed to support the military effort. By the end of 1943, 20 million household Victory Gardens were supplying some 40 percent of the nation's consumption of vegetables.[4]

The generation of Americans who weathered the worst stock market crash in our country's history and emerged as victory gardeners was famously frugal. Wary of the financial sector and industrial power, they turned to self-reliance and the immediate economy they could readily manage in their own households and communities. In many ways, they were not so different from the Jeffersonian farmers of the early 1800s.

But the rising industrial sector, which had gotten a huge boost from the ramp-up to World War II, had ambitious dreams of growth. In 1942, a small group of executives from the nation's leading corporations got together to try to make these dreams a reality. They called their organization the Committee for Economic Development.

Many people have observed the monumental shift that happened in the American economy in the 1970s. Wages stagnated even as productivity continued to grow. Wealth began to concentrate in the hands of the richest 1 percent. Families that had once gotten by on one income suddenly needed two, and they were still going into debt.[5]

Less often discussed is what happened right before 1970: in the preceding decade, the American farm population declined by 26 percent. This was the explicit objective of the Committee for Economic Development, regardless of which political party was in power: use agricultural policy to promote farm consolidation so as to push farmers off the land, create a larger pool of cheap labor, and drive down wages for industrial corporations.[6] Had they presented the bargain this way, of course, the American people would have balked. So in order to persuade Americans to accept a smaller share of the prosperity they were producing, the industrial sector offered them something else, to make it seem that they still had middle-class purchasing power. It offered them cheap goods.

Using a new suite of sophisticated mass marketing techniques, corporate public relations gurus and brand strategists set about reshaping the American producer into the American consumer. Fast food boomed—two-income families working extra hours to make ends meet didn't have time to cook, and inexpensive, calorie-dense comfort food met their needs for both immediate sustenance and a sense of reward for their hard work. Meanwhile, fast-food chains led the way into the new low-wage economy, as the inflation-adjusted value of the minimum wage declined by about 40 percent over the final twenty-five years of the twentieth century. Predictably, their employees didn't like this very much. But in a strategic ploy to pit workers against each other rather than pressuring their greedy employers to share their wealth, the corporations used their massive advertising budgets—as well as their lobbying power—to try to convince Americans to demand lower prices rather than higher wages.[7]

Such was born Americans' fiercely held attachment to cheap consumer goods, particularly cheap food. Transformed from producers into consumers at the same time as their economic status diminished, the American middle class insisted on lower and lower prices, spurred on by corporations like Walmart and McDonald's. With clever brand strategies like the retail giant's Great Value house brand and the fast-food chain's Extra Value menu, these corporations sought to reshape the way Americans thought about value. The word used to mean something about quality, something about an honest transaction and an economy based on fundamental worth. But at Walmart, it just means cheap.

Bombarded as we are with this impoverished notion of value—on billboards, in TV ads, and on the labels of half the things in our kitchen—it's no wonder Americans have gotten in the habit of thinking about how to make food even cheaper so we can pay all the other bills that are stacking up. Despite the fact that we spend less than 10 percent of our income to feed ourselves—half of what our grandparents spent[8]—we are constantly complaining about the high cost of groceries. But the problem with making food cheap so we can pay more for other stuff is that a lot of that other stuff is expensive *because* food is cheap.

Take public assistance programs. Big Food doesn't pay its workers enough to make ends meet, which is why 13 percent of food system workers have to resort to food stamps to feed their own families.[9] So taxpayers effectively subsidize these corporations by making up for the missing wages with $9 billion in public assistance to their workers—just so they can meet basic needs like housing and health care.[10]

Or how about the cost of depleting our natural resources and cleaning up after all the toxic chemicals our cheap food system depends on? One scholar estimates that the public and environmental health losses related to soil erosion in the United States add up to an annual cost of $45 billion. The environmental and health-care costs of US pesticide use? Those set us back another $12 billion. And the annual cost of excessive fertilizer use—application of synthetic nitrogen beyond what plants can use—was estimated by the National Research Council at $2.5 billion.[11]

That last figure may actually be a little low. When Des Moines Water Works sued the drainage districts upstream of its customers for funneling nitrates into their drinking water a few years ago, the lawsuit shined a national spotlight on the cost of cleaning up agricultural pollution. In Iowa alone, experts estimated, solving the water quality problem could cost $1.2 billion annually for several years.[12]

So, as taxpayers, we're spending money to pay for the health-care costs of low-wage food workers. We're also spending money to clean up the public health problems associated with agricultural pollution. And then we're spending *more* money to pay for the health problems associated with this food once it actually makes its way into our bodies. The most commonly cited statistic pegs the annual cost of US obesity at $147 billion, although some experts say it may be as high as $210 billion.[13] Then there's the $116 billion per year we spend on diabetes, plus the hundreds of billions of dollars for diet-related cardiovascular disease and cancer. If you look at the trend lines of US spending on food and health care from the 1960s to today, you can see that they've essentially traded places. In 1960, Americans spent 17.5 percent of their income on food and 5.2 percent on health care. Now we spend 16 percent on health care and a little less than 10 percent on food.[14]

We're robbing Peter to pay Paul. And the worst part is that the Peters in this story are our farmers, our bakers, our neighborhood grocers. The Pauls are pharmaceutical executives and agrichemical tycoons.

For half a century now, this plunder of the American people has been obscured—by corporate advertising, manipulative politics, and the disconnect between our consumer economy and the fundamental economy. But recently, we've reached a morbid tipping point that has made value subtraction very hard to ignore.

At the turn of the millennium, researchers and medical professionals began warning that because of rising obesity rates, children in the United States might not live as long as their parents. In 2014 and 2015, this prediction came true: life expectancy dropped for the first time since the AIDS epidemic in the early 1990s.[15] This modest drop in expected *length* of life grabbed headlines, but behind the scenes, doctors worried even more about what might happen to our national *quality* of life. Given all the technologies we have to keep bodies alive, people suffering from chronic disease are less likely to die young than they are to suffer lengthy, painful declines. The medical community began speaking out. Something had to be done.

As value subtraction comes home to roost in our bodies, it may be that concern for our health is what will finally motivate us all to do something about it. That appears to be the driving factor behind growing markets for organic food and grass-fed beef and declining sales of soda, which recently fell to a thirty-year low.[16]

The case of soda is particularly interesting, as it mirrors in many ways an earlier public health campaign that confronted a powerful industry: tobacco. Taking on tobacco was hard. Smoking permeated American culture, and the industry waged a powerful public relations campaign to combat scientific evidence that it caused lung cancer. Tobacco companies used many of the rhetorical strategies now used by Big Food, accusing government scientists of proliferating a "nanny state" while casting consumption of their products as an exercise of good old American freedom. It took a sustained effort of research, public education, lawsuits, whistle-blowing, and support from medical professionals to turn the tide against tobacco, such that only 15 percent of Americans currently smoke, down from 45 percent in 1954.[17]

Anti-soda campaigns, led by communities hit hard by obesity, have followed a similar multipronged strategy. Public education about the connection between sugar consumption and metabolic disease. Advocacy for changes to federal nutrition guidelines, coupled with changes on the menus of their local schools.[18] And excise taxes on sugary beverages, which have now been passed in four cities in California along with Philadelphia, Seattle, Boulder, and the Navajo Nation (which also taxes other junk foods). Cities with these taxes have seen dramatic declines in soda consumption: in Philly, sales of soda and other sugary drinks went down by 57 percent in the six months after the city's tax went into effect.[19]

But while taxes and public education campaigns were critical to the victory of public health over Big Tobacco, they weren't the whole story. As Michael Pollan pointed out in a 2011 article in *The Nation*,[20] the people who ultimately put a halt to America's smoking addiction were the people who had to pay for it: state governments saddled with Medicaid bills for smoking-related illnesses. They sued. And they won. So now that we have another expensive, preventable public health problem making national news, it begs the question: when will the hospitals and insurers paying for the high cost of cheap food start calling for change?

As it turns out, they already have. In the past decade and a half, over five hundred hospitals have signed the Healthy Food in Health Care Pledge, committing to source food for their cafeterias that is nutritious, environmentally sustainable, and "supportive of human dignity and justice." A similar initiative, the Healthier Hospitals' Healthier Foods Challenge, was launched in 2011 by thirteen of the largest health-care systems in the country. The share of US hospitals participating in one of these two campaigns is now up to 17 percent.[21] Some of them, like St. Luke's in Bethlehem, Pennsylvania, even have organic farms on their campuses—while Kaiser Permanente hosts over fifty farmers markets at its facilities or in nearby communities. Doctors are now beginning to prescribe healthy food instead of just pharmaceuticals.[22]

Schools—which have seen a direct connection between their students' diets, health, and ability to learn—are getting in on the act. Approximately 40,000 school districts participate in the National Farm to School Network, while the most prominent university campaign for better food, the Real Food Challenge, has nudged $60 million in college food spending toward "local, fair, sustainable, and humane food."[23]

As institutions start to drive changes in our food system, there are signs that our culture of cheap food may be shifting as well, particularly among the younger generation. Millennials—those twenty to thirty-six years old who now make up the biggest chunk of the American workforce—are asking more questions about where their food comes from. Three-quarters of them are willing to pay extra for sustainable goods,[24] including food, which is already driving major changes in the industry. Even Rick Schnieders, the former head of food distribution giant Sysco, believes we are seeing the end of the era of "fast, convenient, and cheap." The new watchword, according to Schnieders? Trust.[25]

It's easy to make fun of millennials' foodie obsessions and pooh-pooh their food culture as one big extended episode of *Portlandia*. And it's wise to be skeptical of the idea that dietary fads can solve the larger social problems at the heart of our cheap food crisis. As a nation, we've had a lot of misadventures down that road, from Sylvester Graham's insistence that banning pepper and spices would quell intemperate sexual urges to claims that the Paleo Diet can cure the fatigue experienced by millions of Americans who are working too much and not sleeping enough.

But the good thing about all this conversation about our diet is simply that we're having the conversation. Even Americans' obsession with gluten—while it may be a colossal national misunderstanding—is leading a large number of people to ask important questions about how their food is affecting their health.

The other good news is that, at least when it comes to millennials, renewed interest in where food comes from is not just leading people to become more informed consumers. They're also becoming producers. In 2012, for just the second time in the past century, the US Census of Agriculture showed that the number of farmers under thirty-five years of age was increasing. Compared with their older counterparts, these young farmers are far more likely to raise food organically and sell it locally through community-supported agriculture programs and farmers markets. They're a lot less focused on volume and more focused on quality—in fact, many operate small farms of less than fifty acres.[26] In my neighborhood, some of these young farmers have returned to family farms and started new enterprises, effectively creating small farms within larger ones. Honeybees moved in down the road when one of my neighbors welcomed three kids and a handful of grandkids back to the family farm. Next thing I knew, the local grocery store was carrying honey with my neighbors' name on it. When I drove by, I noticed they'd also planted a vineyard. And another neighbor's high school–aged son was raising goats, with plans to make his future here in Big Sandy, on his family's land.

Even young people who don't farm are shifting from a consumer mindset to an interest in producing more of their own stuff or supporting friends and neighbors who make craft foods and goods. Think about some of those foodie trends lampooned in *Portlandia* episodes: sauerkraut, kimchi, kombucha. These traditional, nutritious ferments are leading the way to a revival of small-scale processing and food preservation. Extension courses like the University of California Master Food Preserver Program and the University of Maryland's "Grow It, Eat It, Preserve It" workshop series have seen a surge of interest.[27] Community education centers like the Institute of Urban Homesteading in Oakland, California, offer workshops in beekeeping, cheese making, herbal medicine preparation, organic gardening, and backyard chicken and goat husbandry. Indigenous leaders from across the country have been rekindling traditional foodways as well, calling for food sovereignty. And many communities have passed cottage food laws to allow small-scale home bakers, preservers, and cheese makers to sell their goods right out of their kitchen.

More important than *what* millennials are doing, however, is *why* they are doing it. In survey after survey, young farmers, gardeners, and eaters say the same thing. It's their values.

As they confront a health crisis, a climate crisis, and a rural economic crisis, I think these young people have gotten wise to the root of the problem. Value is not just about getting things cheaply, as they've been told by Walmart and McDonald's. It's not even really about our stuff. It's about ourselves. Our economy is not just the sum total of our things and their prices; it's a collective decision we all make about what's important: our values. And when we devalue our goods, particularly the most fundamental ones, like food, we devalue ourselves and each other. As we can see from the health problems and social problems we've wrought with cheap food, what we're really talking about here is the value of human life and the value of community.

Since that day in the peach orchard in California when I first realized that agriculture was gearing up for a race to the bottom, I have tried to add value back. I've built up healthy soils on my farm. I've brought jobs back to my rural community. I've done research on ancient grains to understand how the seeds I select impact the health of the people who eat my crop.

I did all of this because I believed it was the right thing to do. But I couldn't have made a living at it were it not for the millions of eaters who demanded healthy, fair, sustainable food. It was these eaters who pulled me into organics, whole grains, and heirloom wheat varieties. By valuing quality, they created markets for farmers like me and businesses like mine. They regenerated thousands of farms and farm towns, supported local bakeries and pasta makers, and brought back forgotten seeds that may hold the key to more nutritious meals. I'll never forget one of my first interactions with such an eater, a woman who walked up to my booth at a trade show in the early 1990s. "Thank you," she said, looking me straight in the eye and shaking my hand heartily, "for growing food for my family." *Thank you?* That is something I never heard as a commodity wheat farmer, and it forever changed the way I saw my farm. From then on, I no longer grew commodities. I only grew food. Good food.

Eaters, I have come to understand, have tremendous power. You can bring large corporations to their knees and force change to extractive business models. You can make family farming viable and challenge farmers to excel as stewards rather than just commodity producers. You can improve your family's well-being and save our health-care system untold billions by demanding more nutritious food. You can even reduce chemical pollution of the earth.

Everyone can be part of this solution. You don't have to be a farmer or a wealthy consumer. Put just one or two more organically grown items in your shopping cart every time you go to the store. Ask your hospital, your local school district, your senior center: Where did that food come from? How was it grown? Are we paying the true cost up front, or are there hidden costs to workers, the environment, and the people who eat it?

It may not seem like a big, dramatic step, but it is through such everyday interactions that we can all set a new standard. For our food. For our treatment of one another and the planet we share. And for the values that give meaning to it all.

Acknowledgments

This book would not have been possible without the encouragement and thoughtful guidance of our agent, Jessica Papin. We have Jessica to thank for putting us in such good hands at Island Press, where President David Miller enthusiastically embraced our vision and masterful editor Emily Turner helped us realize it. We are grateful to everyone else at Island Press who helped bring this book to fruition—Maureen Gately, Sharis Simonian, Elise Ricotta, Julie Marshall, Jaime Jennings, Jason Leppig, Kyler Geoffroy, Rachel Miller, Jen Hawse, and Katharine Sucher—and to copy editor Pat Harris.

University of Montana professor Neva Hassanein offered helpful insight from her research with Kamut International and highlighted key themes that informed our writing. Meanwhile, back in Big Sandy, graphic designer Hilary Page worked heroically to put together the photos and captured a beautiful shot for the jacket cover.

From Bob:

In January 2010, after delivering a guest lecture for an enthusiastic group of college students in Southern Alberta, I was issued a challenge.

My host, Professor Ron Cuthbert, admonished me to write a book of my experiences, charting my philosophy of agriculture and my vision for the future. I began the outline on my drive home, but even with encouragement and suggestions from a host of friends and some professionals, I found the task daunting at best and frustrating at worst. Plagued by a series of false starts, rejected by a favorite publisher, and squeezed by the time press of real life, I let the project drift to the back burner. The manuscript remained untouched and half finished for over a year, until a chance visit with Liz Carlisle at a neighborhood organic farm tour in June 2017. I thought Liz had done a great job with her first book, *Lentil Underground,* and I was confident she could help me with my project. I am thankful she agreed not only to help me but to join with me as a coauthor. She helped me finish in a few months what I had not been able to do in nearly ten years, and I will be forever grateful for her tenacity, hard work, and skill with words and imagery, which have resulted in the book now before you.

In addition to my appreciation to Liz, who helped me *tell* the story, I must add my utmost thanks to so many family members and friends who helped me *live* it—and who have influenced my life in so many ways over the years. (So that you understand my viewpoint of friends: I am of the same mind as Will Rogers, who said, "A stranger is only a friend that I have not met yet.") If I were to give proper credit to all, I would need thank-you footnotes at the bottom of nearly every page of this book, which, quite honestly, would be my preference. But since I cannot double the size of the book in that manner, I want all my friends, mentioned and unmentioned in the book, to know how much I have appreciated your help and friendship over the years. Without all of you, I would not have been able to enjoy my life as I have or to accomplish the deeds recorded in this book. However, there are a few who need to be mentioned by name. They are in four categories—family, teachers, mentors, and business partners—dear friends all.

I must start with my parents, Mack and Dordy Quinn, who guided me from my earliest days and supported and encouraged me throughout my life. During the past forty-eight years, I have my wife, Ann, to thank for her constant (even though sometimes not so enthusiastic) support of my many enterprises and travels throughout the world to promote them. Without her steadfast efforts to raise our five children and help with keeping the farm running in my presence and absence, very few of my efforts with outside enterprises would have been possible. My early love for plants was nourished by my grandfather, Emmet Quinn, and my aunt Pearl Greissinger, and with the loving encouragement of my other grandparents, uncles, aunts, and cousins, I had the support system I needed to mold my formative years in a very positive way. Thank you all!

My science teachers had the biggest influence on the direction of my life's work. Those who influenced me most in high school and college were Mr. Robert Chvilicek in Big Sandy and Dr. Gary Stroble and Dr. Don Mathre in Bozeman. Those three propelled my love of plant science and then taught me the use of the scientific method of investigation and inquiry, which has served me throughout my life of research and observations. I also appreciate all the rest of my teachers who influenced and trained me. Thank you all!

Although my list of mentors and friends who have influenced and helped me is nearly endless, I will name three who have continued to advise and encourage me since we first met over thirty years ago. They have influenced my introduction to, adoption of, and promotion of organic agriculture, which has done more to change the direction of my professional life than anything else. The three I would like to mention who have been friends and advisors since the mid-1980s are Dave Vetter (Nebraska), Thomas Harding (Pennsylvania), and Fred Kirschenmann (North Dakota). Without those three and a host of others, I would not have learned the lessons I needed to lead me to the discoveries described in this writing. Thank you all!

My style of doing business is to find good partners who complement my experience and business philosophy with their own unique qualities. I would also like to pay special tribute to the many employees and interns who have helped me over the years. Good help is hard to find, and I have been blessed with some of the best. Again, the list of such partners and employees is too long for me to mention them all and express my sincere appreciation individually. There have been a lot of enterprises and projects over the past forty-five years. However, I will at least mention my first business partner, as well as my longest one. Randy Nieffenegger and I met at UC Davis and started Quiger Laboratory together in nearby Woodland, in the old Porter Building on Main Street around 1973. It was my first business experience and my steepest learning curve, and I could not have done it without him. My longest-term business partner is Mark Callebert of Belgium. We first starting working together to bring the Kamut brand to Europe in 1991, and we have worked on that project together ever since. I am most grateful to him for his insight in helping to work through the many challenges we have had over the years. Again, to those business associates named and unnamed in the book, here in Big Sandy and beyond, I thank you all!

Finally, to my readers: I thank you for taking the time to read this book. I hope it has increased your understanding of the past and present of agriculture in the United States as well as your hope and vision for food and health in the future. And I hope you enjoyed reading this book as much as I have enjoyed living it. Thank you all!

Your friend—Bob

From Liz:

First, I want to thank Bob Quinn for inviting me to collaborate on this project. It's truly an honor, and I am deeply grateful for Bob's insight, humor, and unfailingly gracious attitude.

A number of fellow writers and scholars generously took time away from their own work to read early drafts of the manuscript and provide helpful feedback that improved the final version: Maywa Montenegro, Emily Polk, Rob Jackson, Richard Nevle, Lauren Oakes, Russ Carpenter, Shannon Switzer Swanson, and Bruce Maxwell.

My mentors Michael Pollan and Tom Hayden provided critical guidance and encouragement in the early stages of this project, and my students and colleagues at Stanford University were a continual source of inspiration and support.

My parents, Lynne and Ray Carlisle, hosted me for a short-notice writing retreat that got us most of the way through the first draft.

Though I've never met anybody at Trint, I want to give them all a hug for creating a digital transcription tool that made it possible for us to meet our deadlines.

I cannot adequately express my gratitude to Patrick Archie, my partner in life and agroecology, for all the many ways in which he contributes to my happiness and my thinking. The seeds of this book were planted in his nurturing presence, as a conversation on a farm tour, and he has been encouraging them along ever since.

Notes

Prologue

1. J. L. Fox, "Wind Is Driving Energy Development in Montana," *Bozeman (MT) Daily Chronicle*, 14 March 2015, www.bozemandailychronicle.com /opinions/guest_columnists/wind-is-driving-energy-development-in -montana/article_e5bad960-0792-5394-b131-abf/40ff429c.html.

Introduction: Food on the Cheap

1. E. Barclay, "Your Grandparents Spent More of Their Money on Food than You Do," *The Salt*, National Public Radio, 2 March 2015, www.npr .org/sections/thesalt/2015/03/02/389578089/your-grandparents-spent -more-of-their-money-on-food-than-you-do.

2. Our World in Data, https://ourworldindata.org/employment-in-agricul ture.

3. J. Berry, "Statistics and Facts about Type 2 Diabetes," *Medical News Today*, 12 June 2018, www.medicalnewstoday.com/articles/318472.php.

4. S. Ro, "Chart of the Day: The Stunning Rise of Disability, Food Stamp, and Welfare Benefits," *Business Insider*, 6 February 2014, www.business insider.com/chart-disability-food-stamps-welfare-2014-2.

5. R. Laudan, *Cuisine and Empire: Cooking in World History* (Berkeley: University of California Press, 2013), e-book, p. 126.

6. M. Pollan, *Cooked: A Natural History of Transformation* (New York: Penguin Books, 2013), p. 254.

7. A. Bobrow-Strain, *White Bread: A Social History of the Store-Bought Loaf* (Boston: Beacon Press, 2012), p. 111.

8. Pollan, *Cooked*, p. 226.

9. World Health Organization, International Agency for Research on Cancer, "IARC Monograph on Glyphosate," 3 January 2013, www.iarc.fr/en /media-centre/iarcnews/2016/glyphosate_IARC2016.php.

10. C. Jones and R. Engel, "Soil Acidification: Causes, Management, and Research, Chouteau County," Montana State University, 22 March 2017, http://landresources.montana.edu/soilfertility/documents/PDF/pres/Soil AcidityChouteauMar2017.pdf.

11. National Oceanic and Atmospheric Administration (NOAA), "Gulf of Mexico 'Dead Zone' Is the Largest Ever Measured," 2 August 2017, www .noaa.gov/media-release/gulf-of-mexico-dead-zone-is-largest-ever-measured; NOAA, National Ocean Service, "What Is a Dead Zone?," https://ocean service.noaa.gov/facts/deadzone.html.

12. P. McMichael, "A Food Regime Analysis of the 'World Food Crisis,'" *Agriculture and Human Values* 26 (2009): 282.

13. N. Gilbert, "One-Third of Our Greenhouse Gas Emissions Come from Agriculture," *Nature*, 31 October 2012, www.nature.com/news/one-third -of-our-greenhouse-gas-emissions-come-from-agriculture-1.11708.

14. M. Carolan, *The Real Cost of Cheap Food* (New York: Earthscan, 2011).

15. J. L. Zagorsky and P. Smith, "Do Poor People Eat More Junk Food than Wealthier Americans?," *The Conversation*, 13 June 2017, http://theconver sation.com/do-poor-people-eat-more-junk-food-than-wealthier-americans -79154.

16. D. Miller, *Farmacology: Total Health from the Ground Up* (New York: William Morrow, 2013).

17. Organic Trade Association, www.ota.com/resources/market-analysis.

18. Stone Barns Center for Food and Agriculture et al., "Back to Grass: The Market Potential for U.S. Grassfed Beef," April 2017, www.stonebarns center.org/wp-content/uploads/2017/10/Grassfed_Full_v2.pdf.

19. Specialty Coffee Association of America, "Specialty Coffee Facts and Figures," updated March 2012, www.scaa.org/PDF/resources/facts-and-fig ures.pdf.

20. International Panel of Experts on Sustainable Food Systems (IPES-Food), "From Uniformity to Diversity: A Paradigm Shift from Industrial Agriculture to Diversified Agroecological Systems," June 2016, www.ipes-food .org/images/Reports/UniformityToDiversity_FullReport.pdf.

Chapter 1: Roots and Growth

1. D. Hofsommer, "Hill's Dream Realized: The Burlington Northern's Eight-Decade Gestation," *Pacific Northwest Quarterly* 79, no. 4 (1988): 138–46.

2. T. A. Lyson, *Civic Agriculture: Reconnecting Farm, Food, and Community* (Medford, MA: Tufts University Press, 2004), p. 21.

3. W. Hauter, *Foodopoly: The Battle over the Future of Food and Farming in America* (New York: New Press, 2012), p. 21.

4. C. Gibson, "American Demographic History Chartbook: 1790 to 2010," 2010, figure 2-2, http://demographicchartbook.com/wp-content/uploads /2015/11/Gibson-DemographicChartbook.pdf.

5. Motorola Inc., advertisement in *Farm Journal*, May 1951, https://reposi tory.duke.edu/dc/adaccess/TV0232.

Chapter 2: Better Farming through Chemistry?

1. US Department of the Interior, Bureau of Reclamation, "Montana Bald Eagle Management Plan," July 1994, www.fws.gov/montanafieldoffice /Endangered_Species/Recovery_and_Mgmt_Plans/Montana_Bald_Eagle _mgmt_plan.pdf.

2. US Department of Agriculture, Economic Research Service, "Recent Trends in GE Adoption," 12 July 2017, www.ers.usda.gov/data-products /adoption-of-genetically-engineered-crops-in-the-us/recent-trends-in-ge -adoption.aspx; J. Fernandez Cornejo, S. J. Wechsler, and D. Milkove, "The Adoption of Genetically Engineered Alfalfa, Canola, and Sugarbeets in the United States," November 2016, US Department of Agriculture, Economic Research Service Economic Information Bulletin No. EIB-163, www.ers.usda.gov/publications/pub-details/?pubid=81175.

3. D. Hakim, "Monsanto's Weed Killer, Dicamba, Divides Farmers," *New York Times*, 21 September 2017, https://mobile.nytimes.com/2017/09/21 /business/monsanto-dicamba-weed-killer.html.

Chapter 3: Beyond Commodities

1. T. A. Lyson, *Civic Agriculture: Reconnecting Farm, Food, and Community* (Medford, MA: Tufts University Press, 2004), p. 44.

2. W. Hauter, *Foodopoly: The Battle over the Future of Food and Farming in America* (New York: New Press, 2012), pp. 14, 20.

3. M. Pollan, *The Omnivore's Dilemma: A Natural History of Four Meals* (New York: Penguin Books, 2006), pp. 51–53.

4. Hauter, *Foodopoly*, pp. 22, 23.

5. Hauter, *Foodopoly*, p. 22.

6. Lyson, *Civic Agriculture*, p. 20.

7. Hauter, *Foodopoly*, p. 24.

8. M. Carolan, *The Real Cost of Cheap Food* (New York: Earthscan, 2011), p. 167.

9. Carolan, *Real Cost of Cheap Food*, p. 168.

10. Lyson, *Civic Agriculture*, p. 32.

11. Hauter, *Foodopoly*, p. 24.

12. F. Jabr, "Bread Is Broken," *New York Times Magazine*, 29 October 2015, www.nytimes.com/2015/11/01/magazine/bread-is-broken.html.

13. N. Myhrvold and F. Migoya, *Modernist Bread*, vol. 1, *History and Fundamentals* (Bellevue, WA: The Cooking Lab, 2017).

14. A. Bobrow-Strain, *White Bread: A Social History of the Store-Bought Loaf* (Boston: Beacon Press, 2012), p. 78.

15. M. Pollan, *Cooked: A Natural History of Transformation* (New York: Penguin Books, 2013), p. 254.

16. Pollan, *Cooked*, p. 253.

17. Pollan, *Cooked*, p. 254.

18. Jabr, "Bread Is Broken."

19. Pollan, *Cooked*, p. 259.

20. L. J. Davenport, "The History, Natural History, and Biogeography of Graham Bread," *Alabama Heritage* 104 (2012): 53–54; D. Roth, "America's Fascination with Nutrition," *Food Review* 23, no. 1 (2000): 32–37.

21. M. C. Neely, "Embodied Politics: Antebellum Vegetarianism and the Dietary Economy of Walden," *American Literature* 85, no. 1 (2013): 43.

22. Roth, "America's Fascination with Nutrition."

23. H. Levenstein, *Paradox of Plenty: A Social History of Eating in Modern America* (Berkeley: University of California Press, 2003), p. 65.

24. H. W. Wiley, "The End of the Bleached Flour Case," *Good Housekeeping*, June 1914, p. 832, cited in A. Bobrow-Strain, "Kills a Body Twelve Ways: Bread Fear and the Politics of 'What to Eat?,'" *Gastronomica: The Journal of Critical Food Studies* 7, no. 3 (Summer 2007): 45–52, https://doi.org/10.1525/gfc.2007.7.3.45.

25. Levenstein, *Paradox of Plenty*, p. 68.

26. W. Shurtleff and A. Aoyagi, *History of Erewhon—Natural Foods Pioneer in the United States (1966–2011): Extensively Annotated Bibliography and Sourcebook* (Lafayette, CA: Soyinfo Center, 2011), www.soyinfocenter.com/pdf/142/Erewhon2.pdf, p. 10.

27. Levenstein, *Paradox of Plenty*, p. 184.

28. Levenstein, *Paradox of Plenty*, p. 184.

29. Levenstein, *Paradox of Plenty*, pp. 185, 193.

30. F. Fabricant, "The Whole-Grain Movement Carries On," *New York Times*, 13 June 1984, www.nytimes.com/1984/06/13/garden/the-whole-grain -movement-carries-on.html.

31. F. Magdoff and H. van Es, *Building Soils for Better Crops*, 3rd ed. (Beltsville, MD: Sustainable Agriculture Research and Education, 2009), www .sare.org/Learning-Center/Books/Building-Soils-for-Better-Crops-3rd -Edition/Text-Version/The-Living-Soil/Soil-Microorganisms.

32. D. R. Montgomery, *Growing a Revolution: Bringing Our Soil Back to Life* (New York: W. W. Norton, 2017), p. 49.

Chapter 4: Going Organic

1. I wasn't alone. Data from the USDA's Economic Research Service show that in 1984, Montana farmers paid just over $157 million for pesticides, fertilizer, lime, and soil conditioner. Their net income that year? A loss of $112 million. And their government payments: $239 million. Without the federal subsidy, you'd think farmers might have learned their lesson and tried to lower their input costs. But in 1985, Montana farmers spent another $134 million on chemicals. That year they lost a whopping $333 million: the worst year of the 1980s. But again, Uncle Sam helped them cover the chemical bill, to the tune of over $220 million. US Department of Agriculture, Economic Research Service, "Farm Income and Wealth Statistics, Value Added Years by State," 2018, https://data.ers.usda.gov/reports .aspx?ID=17830#Pa3316c27a2b94883b3008821125d2680_8_110iT0R0x26.

2. Sustainable Agriculture Research and Education, "2016 Cover Crop Survey Analysis," www.sare.org/Learning-Center/From-the-Field/North -Central-SARE-From-the-Field/2016-Cover-Crop-Survey-Analysis.

3. D. Bigelow, "A Primer on Land Use in the United States," US Department of Agriculture, Economic Research Service, 4 December 2017, www.ers.usda.gov/amber-waves/2017/december/a-primer-on-land-use-in -the-united-states/.

Chapter 5: King Tut's Wheat

1. M. Pollan, *Cooked: A Natural History of Transformation* (New York: Penguin Books, 2013), p. 265.

2. Pollan, *Cooked*, pp. 258–59.

3. Pollan, *Cooked*, pp. 261–62.

Chapter 6: Growing Partners

1. F. Mayer et al., "Use of Polymorphisms in the γ-Gliadin Gene of Spelt and Wheat as a Tool for Authenticity Control," *Journal of Agricultural and Food Chemistry* 60, no. 6 (2012): 1350–57, https://doi.org/10.1021/jf203945d; J. Bönick, G. Huschek, and H. M. Rawel, "Determination of Wheat, Rye, and Spelt Authenticity in Bread by Targeted Peptide Biomarkers," *Journal of Food Composition and Analysis* 58 (May 2017): 82–91, https://doi.org/10.1016/j.jfca.2017.01.019.

2. US Department of Agriculture, Economic Research Service, "Recent Trends in GE Adoption," 12 July 2017, www.ers.usda.gov/data-products/adoption-of-genetically-engineered-crops-in-the-us/recent-trends-in-ge-adoption.aspx.

3. B. Spiegel, "Hybrid Wheat's Comeback," *Successful Farming*, 11 March 2013, www.agriculture.com/crops/wheat/technology/hybrid-wheats-come back_147-ar30398.

4. T. Lutey, "The Accidental Release of Forbidden GMO Wheat in Huntley Could Have Been Catastrophic," *Billings (MT) Gazette*, 28 August 2016, http://billingsgazette.com/news/state-and-regional/montana/the-accidental-release-of-forbidden-gmo-wheat-in-huntley-could/article_5d72d942-1d21-5f87-9df2-85a72bb755bd.html.

Chapter 7: A Cowboy in Europe

1. They would, of course, get in on VHS later, but not before losing their shirt on Betamax. J. Lardner, *Fast Forward: Hollywood, the Japanese, and the Onslaught of the VCR* (New York: W. W. Norton, 1987).

2. T. Mitchell, *Rule of Experts: Egypt, Techno-Politics, Modernity* (Berkeley: University of California Press, 2002), chap. 1.

3. Mitchell, *Rule of Experts*, p. 20.

4. Mitchell, *Rule of Experts*, p. 20.

5. C. L. Weber and H. S. Matthews, "Food-Miles and the Relative Climate Impacts of Food Choices in the United States," *Environmental Science and Technology* 42, no. 10 (2008): 3508–13, https://doi.org/10.1021/es702969f.

6. H. Friedmann, "The Political Economy of Food: The Rise and Fall of the Postwar International Food Order," *American Journal of Sociology* 88 (1982): S248–86, https://doi.org/10.1086/649258.

7. C. Reichelt, "King Tut Wheat, 'Corn' of Egypt's Ancients," *Great Falls (MT) Tribune*, 7 June 1964.

Chapter 8: Creating a New Standard

1. M. A. Haedicke, *Organizing Organic: Conflict and Compromise in an Emerging Market* (Stanford, CA: Stanford University Press, 2016), p. 76.

2. S. Zavestoski, S. Shulman, and D. Schlosberg, "Democracy and the Environment on the Internet: Electronic Citizen Participation in Regulatory Rulemaking," *Science, Technology, & Human Values* 31, no. 4 (2006): 385, https://doi.org/10.1177/0162243906287543.

3. Haedicke, *Organizing Organic*, pp. 75–76.

4. Zavestoski, Shulman, and Schlosberg, "Democracy and the Environment," p. 394.

5. Haedicke, *Organizing Organic*, p. 76.

6. M. Nestle, *Food Politics: How the Food Industry Influences Nutrition and Health*, 2nd ed. (Berkeley: University of California Press, 2013).

7. E. Grossman, "A Shocking Number of Chemical Products Are Banned in Europe but Safe in the US," *Ensia/Business Insider*, 10 June 2014, www.businessinsider.com/products-banned-in-europe but safe-in-us-2014-6.

8. A. E. M. Hess, "These 10 Companies Control the World's Food," *Huffington Post*, 18 August 2014, www.huffingtonpost.com/2014/08/17/companies-control-food_n_5684782.html.

9. "Philip H. Howard," https://philhoward.net/.

10. J. M. MacDonald, "Mergers and Competition in Seed and Agricultural Chemical Markets," US Department of Agriculture, Economic Research Service, 3 April 2017, www.ers.usda.gov/amber-waves/2017/april/mergers-and-competition-in-seed-and-agricultural-chemical-markets/.

11. T. Philpott, "Monsanto Now Belongs to Bayer," *Mother Jones*, 13 September 2016, www.motherjones.com/environment/2016/09/whoa-monsanto-about-get-swallowed-german-giant-bayer/#.

12. W. Hauter, *Foodopoly: The Battle over the Future of Food and Farming in America* (New York: New Press, 2012), p. 160.

13. Hauter, *Foodopoly*, p. 173.

14. Hauter, *Foodopoly*, p. 192.

15. Hauter, *Foodopoly*, p. 220.

16. Hauter, *Foodopoly*, p. 173.

17. Friends of the Earth Europe, "Agrifood Atlas: Facts and Figures about the Corporations That Control What We Eat," p. 26, www.foeeurope.org/sites/default/files/agriculture/2017/agrifood_atlas.pdf.

18. P. Howard, "AFHVS 2016 Presidential Address: Decoding Diversity in

the Food System: Wheat and Bread in North America," *Agriculture and Human Values* 33, no. 4 (December 2016): 953–60, https://doi.org/10.1007/s10460-016-9727-y.

19. T. A. Lyson, *Civic Agriculture: Reconnecting Farm, Food, and Community* (Medford, MA: Tufts University Press, 2004), p. 58.

20. K. Karson, "Trump USDA Withdraws Animal Welfare Regulation for Organic Farms, Sparking Backlash," ABC News, 14 March 2018, https://abcnews.go.com/US/trump-usda-withdraws-animal-welfare-regulation-organic-farms/story?id=53745900.

Chapter 9: The Value of Limits

1. J. Erbentraut, "Hunger in Rural America Is Less Visible, but Just as Pressing," *Huffington Post*, 12 May 2017, www.huffingtonpost.com/entry/rural-communities-hunger-rates_us_59148645e4b030d4f1f09941.

2. P. L. Brown et al., "Saline-Seep Diagnosis, Control, and Reclamation," US Department of Agriculture Conservation Research Report No. 30, 1982, p. 4, www.nrcs.usda.gov/Internet/FSE_DOCUMENTS/stelprdb 1044791.pdf.

3. J. A. Widtsoe, *Dry-Farming: A System of Agriculture for Countries under a Low Rainfall* (New York: Macmillan, 1913).

4. B. Barth, "When the Well Runs Dry, Try Dry Farming," *Modern Farmer*, 10 July 2014, http://modernfarmer.com/2014/07/well-runs-dry-try-dry-farming/.

5. California Ag Water Stewardship Initiative, "Dry Farming," http://agwa terstewards.org/practices/dry_farming/.

6. H. Cooley et al., "Global Water Governance in the Twenty-First Century," in *The World's Water*, vol. 8, ed. P. H. Gleick (Washington, DC: Island Press/Center for Resource Economics, 2014), pp. 1–18.

7. Y. Wada et al., "Global Depletion of Groundwater Resources," *Geophysical Research Letters* 37, no. 20 (2010): 1–5, https://doi.org/10.1029/2010GL044571.

8. Intergovernmental Panel on Climate Change, "Climate Change and Water," IPCC Technical Paper 6, ed. B. C. Bates et al., June 2008, p. 7, https://drive.google.com/file/d/0B1gFp6Ioo3akcFFFeGRRVFNYM0E/view.

9. Cooley et al., "Global Water Governance."

10. W. M. Jarrell and R. B. Beverly, "The Dilution Effect in Plant Nutrition Studies," *Advances in Agronomy* 34 (1981): 197–224, https://doi.org/10.1016/S0065-2113(08)60887-1.

11. Charles Benbrook, email message to Liz Carlisle, 20 November 2017.

12. Benbrook, email to Carlisle, 20 November 2017; C. Benbrook, "The Impacts of Yield on Nutritional Quality: Lessons from Organic Farming," *HortScience* 44, no. 1 (2009): 12–14; M. Barański et al., "Higher Antioxidant and Lower Cadmium Concentrations and Lower Incidence of Pesticide Residues in Organically Grown Crops: A Systematic Literature Review and Meta-analyses," *British Journal of Nutrition* 112, no. 5 (2014): 794–811, https://doi.org/10.1017/S0007114514001366.

13. D. R. Davis, M. D. Epp, and H. D. Riordan, "Changes in USDA Food Composition Data for 43 Garden Crops, 1950 to 1999," *Journal of the American College of Nutrition* 23, no. 6 (2004): 669–82, https://doi.org/10.1080/07315724.2004.10719409.

14. D. R. Davis, "Declining Fruit and Vegetable Nutrient Composition: What Is the Evidence?," *HortScience* 44, no. 1 (2009): 15–19; K. M. Murphy, P. G. Reeves, and S. S. Jones, "Relationship between Yield and Mineral Nutrient Concentrations in Historical and Modern Spring Wheat Cultivars," *Euphytica* 163, no. 3 (2008): 381–90, https://doi.org/10.1007/s10681-008-9681-x.

Chapter 10: Taste of Place

1. A. B. Trubek, *The Taste of Place: A Cultural Journey into Terroir* (Berkeley: University of California Press, 2008), p. xv.

2. Trubek, *Taste of Place*, p. 36.

3. Trubek, *Taste of Place*, p. 49.

4. Trubek, *Taste of Place*, p. 131.

5. R. Patel, A. Kinezuka, and M. Montenegro, "International Trade, Corporate Power, and Food Sovereignty," in *Bite Back: Winning Victories for a New Food Democracy*, ed. K. De Master and S. Jayaraman (Berkeley: University of California Press, 2019).

6. E. Ptak, "Marin Agricultural Land Trust: Preserving Marin County Farmland," *Civil Eats*, 7 August 2008, https://civileats.com/2008/08/07/marin-agricultural-land-trustpreserving-marin-county-farmland/.

7. Trubek, *Taste of Place*, p. 194.

Chapter 11: Recycling Energy

1. M. C. Heller and G. A. Keoleian, "Life Cycle–Based Sustainability Indicators for Assessment of the U.S. Food System," Center for Sustainable Systems Report No. CSS00-04 (Ann Arbor: University of Michigan

School of Natural Resources and Environment, 6 December 2000), p. 42, http://css.umich.edu/sites/default/files/css_doc/CSS00-04.pdf.

2. Heller and Keoleian, "Sustainability Indicators."

3. D. Pimentel, "Impacts of Organic Farming on the Efficiency of Energy Use in Agriculture: An Organic Center State of Science Review" (Foster, RI: The Organic Center, August 2006), p. 5, www.organic-center.org /reportfiles/ENERGY_SSR.pdf.

4. International Panel of Experts on Sustainable Food Systems (IPES-Food), "From Uniformity to Diversity: A Paradigm Shift from Industrial Agriculture to Diversified Agroecological Systems," June 2016, www.ipes-food .org/images/Reports/UniformityToDiversity_FullReport.pdf.

5. D. Pimentel and W. Dazhong, "Technological Changes in Energy Use in U.S. Agricultural Production," in *Agroecology*, ed. C. R. Carroll, J. H. Vandermeer, and P. Rosset (New York: McGraw-Hill, 1990).

6. Pimentel, "Impacts of Organic Farming," p. 1.

7. Pimentel, "Impacts of Organic Farming," p. 1.

8. M. Pollan, *The Omnivore's Dilemma: A Natural History of Four Meals* (New York: Penguin Books, 2006), pp. 113–14.

9. Judith Gap Wind Farm dedication, video, 1 October 2005.

10. J. A. Blize, "The Power of Wind: A Citizen's Guide to Wind Development in Montana," Temple University School of Environmental Design, 2010, www.wccapa.org/wp-content/uploads/2011/06/Wind-Develop ment-in-MT.pdf.

11. Associated Press, "Judith Gap Wind Farm a Success," *Billings (MT) Gazette*, 20 November 2006, http://billingsgazette.com/news/state-and -regional/montana/judith-gap-wind-farm-a-success/article_81533d3d -d0c7-5495-9f28-c371ebe7faa3.html.

12. J. L. Fox, "Wind Is Driving Energy Development in Montana," *Bozeman (MT) Daily Chronicle*, 14 March 2015, www.bozemandailychronicle.com /opinions/guest_columnists/wind-is-driving-energy-development-in -montana/article_e5bad960-0792-5394-b131-abf740ff429c.html.

Chapter 12: Bringing Rural Jobs Back

1. B. Thiede et al., "The Divide between Rural and Urban America, in 6 Charts," *U.S. News & World Report*, 20 March 2017, www.usnews.com /news/national-news/articles/2017-03-20/6-charts-that-illustrate-the -divide-between-rural-and-urban-america.

2. Thiede et al., "Divide between Rural and Urban America."

3. D. Weingarten, "Why Are America's Farmers Killing Themselves in Record Numbers?," *Guardian* (US edition), 6 December 2017, www.the guardian.com/us-news/2017/dec/06/why-are-americas-farmers-killing -themselves-in-record-numbers.

4. E. C. Jaenicke, "U.S. Organic Hotspots and Their Benefit to Local Economies," Organic Trade Association, 2016, www.ota.com/hotspots.

5. M. Carolan, *The Real Cost of Cheap Food* (New York: Earthscan, 2011), pp. 167–68.

6. B. B. R. Jablonski et al., "Do Local Food Markets Support Profitable Farms and Ranches?," *Union of Concerned Scientists Blog*, 26 April 2018, https://blog.ucsusa.org/science-blogger/do-local-food-markets-support -profitable-farms-and-ranches.

Chapter 13: The Gluten Mystery

1. M. Nestle, *Food Politics: How the Food Industry Influences Nutrition and Health*, 2nd ed. (Berkeley: University of California Press, 2013).

2. K. C. Maki and A. K. Phillips, "Dietary Substitutions for Refined Carbohydrate That Show Promise for Reducing Risk of Type 2 Diabetes in Men and Women," *Journal of Nutrition* 145, no. 1 (2015): 159–63S, https://doi.org/10.3945/jn.114.195149.

3. R. Giacco et al., "Whole Grain Intake in Relation to Body Weight: From Epidemiological Evidence to Clinical Trials," *Nutrition, Metabolism & Cardiovascular Diseases* 21, no. 12 (2011): 901–8, https://doi.org/10.1016 /j.numecd.2011.07.003.

4. N. R. Sahyoun et al., "Whole-Grain Intake Is Inversely Associated with the Metabolic Syndrome and Mortality in Older Adults," *American Journal of Clinical Nutrition* 83, no. 1 (2006): 124–31, https://doi.org/10 .1093/ajcn/83.1.124; A. Gil, R. M. Ortega, and J. Maldonado, "Whole-grain Cereals and Bread: A Duet of the Mediterranean Diet for the Prevention of Chronic Diseases," *Public Health Nutrition* 14, no. 12A (2011): 2316–22, https://doi.org/10.1017/S1368980011002576.

5. M. Pollan, *Cooked: A Natural History of Transformation* (New York: Penguin Books, 2013), p. 270.

6. J. Slavin, "Why Whole Grains Are Protective: Biological Mechanisms," *Proceedings of the Nutrition Society* 62, no. 1 (2003): 129–34, https://doi .org/10.1079/PNS2002221.

7. K. K. Adom and R. H. Liu, "Antioxidant Activity of Grains," *Journal of Agricultural and Food Chemistry* 50, no. 21 (2002): 6182–87, https://doi

.org/10.1021/jf0205099; R. H. Liu, "Potential Synergy of Phytochemicals in Cancer Prevention: Mechanism of Action," *Journal of Nutrition* 134, no. 12 (2004): 3479–85S, https://doi.org/10.1093/jn/134.12.3479S.

8. Pollan, *Cooked,* pp. 261–62.

9. A. Carnevali et al., "Role of Kamut® Brand Khorasan Wheat in the Counteraction of Non-celiac Wheat Sensitivity and Oxidative Damage," *Food Research International* 63, part B (September 2014): 218–26, https://doi.org/10.1016/j.foodres.2014.01.065.

10. F. Penagini et al., "Gluten-Free Diet in Children: An Approach to a Nutritionally Adequate and Balanced Diet," *Nutrients* 5, no. 11 (2013): 4553–65, https://doi.org/10.3390/nu5114553.

11. R. M. Quinn, "Kamut®: Ancient Grain, New Cereal," in *Perspectives on New Crops and New Uses,* ed. J. Janick (Alexandria, VA: ASHS Press, 1999), pp. 182–83.

12. A. Gianotti et al., "Role of Cereal Type and Processing in Whole Grain In Vivo Protection from Oxidative Stress," *Frontiers in Bioscience* 16 (2011): 1609–18.

13. S. Benedetti et al., "Counteraction of Oxidative Damage in the Rat Liver by an Ancient Grain (Kamut Brand Khorasan Wheat)," *Nutrition* 28, no. 4 (2012): 436–41, https://doi.org/10.1016/j.nut.2011.08.006.

14. P. Hunter, "The Inflammation Theory of Disease," *EMBO Reports* 13, no. 11 (2012): 968–70, https://doi.org/10.1038/embor.2012.142.

15. Carnevali et al., "Role of Kamut® Brand Khorasan Wheat."

Chapter 14: Food as Medicine

1. F. Sofi et al., 2013. "Characterization of Khorasan Wheat (Kamut) and Impact of a Replacement Diet on Cardiovascular Risk Factors: Cross-over Dietary Intervention Study," *European Journal of Clinical Nutrition* 67, no. 2 (2013): 190–95.

2. "Inflammation," *Encyclopaedia Brittanica,* 2018, www.britannica.com/science/inflammation.

3. F. Sofi et al., "Effect of *Triticum turgidum* Subsp. *turanicum* Wheat on Irritable Bowel Syndrome: A Double-Blinded Randomised Dietary Intervention Trial," *British Journal of Nutrition* 111, no. 11 (2014): 1992–99, https://doi.org/10.1017/S000711451400018X.

4. T. G. Dinan et al., "Enhanced Cholinergic-Mediated Increase in the Pro-inflammatory Cytokine IL-6 in Irritable Bowel Syndrome: Role of

Muscarinic Receptors," *American Journal of Gastroenterology* 103, no. 10 (2008): 2570, http://dx.doi.org/10.1111/j.1572-0241.2008.01871.x.

5. M. Camilleri, "Peripheral Mechanisms in Irritable Bowel Syndrome," *New England Journal of Medicine* 367, no. 17 (2012): 1626–35, https://doi.org/10.1056/NEJMra1207068; A. C. Ford and N. J. Talley, "Irritable Bowel Syndrome," *British Medical Journal* 345 (2012): e5836, https://doi.org/10.1136/bmj.e5836.

6. A. Carroccio, G. Rini, and P. Mansueto, "Non-Celiac Wheat Sensitivity Is a More Appropriate Label than Non-Celiac Gluten Sensitivity," *Gastroenterology* 146, no. 1 (2014): 320–21, https://doi.org/10.1053/j.gastro.2013.08.061.

7. A. Whittaker et al., "An Organic Khorasan Wheat–Based Replacement Diet Improves Risk Profile of Patients with Acute Coronary Syndrome: A Randomized Crossover Trial," *Nutrients* 7, no. 5 (2015): 3401–15, https://doi.org/10.3390/nu7053401.

8. F. Sofi et al., "Mediterranean Diet and Health Status: An Updated Meta-analysis and a Proposal for a Literature-Based Adherence Score," *Public Health Nutrition* 17, no. 12 (2014): 2769–82, https://doi.org/10.1017/S1368980013003169; S. Yusuf et al., "Effect of Potentially Modifiable Risk Factors Associated with Myocardial Infarction in 52 Countries (the INTERHEART Study): Case-Control Study," *The Lancet* 364, no. 9438 (2004): 937–52, https://doi.org/10.1016/S0140-6736(04)17018-9.

9. S. C. Port et al., "Blood Glucose: A Strong Risk Factor for Mortality in Nondiabetic Patients with Cardiovascular Disease," *American Heart Journal* 150, no. 2 (2005): 209–14, https://doi.org/10.1016/j.ahj.2004.09.031.

10. D. Esposito et al., "A Journey into a Mediterranean Diet and Type 2 Diabetes: A Systematic Review with Meta-analyses," *BMJ Open* 5, no. 8 (2015): e008222, http://dx.doi.org/10.1136/bmjopen-2015-008222.

11. Ł. Czyżewska-Majchrzak et al., "The Use of Low-Carbohydrate Diet in Type 2 Diabetes—Benefits and Risks," *Annals of Agricultural and Environmental Medicine* 21, no. 2 (2014): 320–26, https://doi.org/10.5604/1232-1966.1108597.

12. A. Whittaker et al., "A Khorasan Wheat–Based Replacement Diet Improves Risk Profile of Patients with Type 2 Diabetes Mellitus (T2DM): A Randomized Crossover Trial," *European Journal of Nutrition* 56, no. 3 (2017): 1191–1200, https://doi.org/10.1007/s00394-016-1168-2.

13. M. Dinu et al., "A Khorasan Wheat–Based Replacement Diet Improves Risk Profile of Patients with Nonalcoholic Fatty Liver Disease (NAFLD):

A Randomized Clinical Trial," *Journal of the American College of Nutrition* 37, no. 6 (2018): 508–14, https://doi.org/10.1080/07315724.2018 .1445047.

14. G. Dinelli et al., "Determination of Phenolic Compounds in Modern and Old Varieties of Durum Wheat Using Liquid Chromatography Coupled with Time-of-Flight Mass Spectrometry," *Journal of Chromatography A* 1216, no. 43 (2009): 7229–40, https://doi.org/10.1016/j.chroma.2009 .08.041.

15. D. T. Saa et al., "Impact of Kamut® Khorasan on Gut Microbiota and Metabolome in Healthy Volunteers," *Food Research International* 63, part B (2014): 227–32, https://doi.org/10.1016/j.foodres.2014.04.005.

16. A. Di Loreto et al., "Nutritional and Nutraceutical Aspects of KAMUT® Khorasan Wheat Grown during the Last Two Decades," *Journal of Agricultural Science* 155, no. 6 (2017): 954–65, https://doi.org/10.1017 /S002185961700003X.

17. For example, K. M. Murphy, P. G. Reeves, and S. S. Jones, "Relationship between Yield and Mineral Nutrient Concentrations in Historical and Modern Spring Wheat Cultivars," *Euphytica* 163, no. 3 (2008): 381–90, https://doi.org/10.1007/s10681-008-9681-x.

18. P. Matson, W. C. Clark, and K. Andersson, *Pursuing Sustainability: A Guide to the Science and Practice* (Princeton, NJ: Princeton University Press, 2016).

19. World Health Organization (WHO), "The Double Burden of Malnutrition: Policy Brief," WHO/NMH/NHD/17.3, 2017, www.who.int /nutrition/publications/doubleburdenmalnutrition-policybrief/en/; see also WHO, "Double Burden of Malnutrition," www.who.int/nutrition /double-burden-malnutrition/en/.

20. Center for Science in the Public Interest, "Why Good Nutrition Is Important," https://cspinet.org/eating-healthy/why-good-nutrition-important.

21. M. Pollan, "Big Food vs. Big Insurance," *New York Times*, 9 September 2009, www.nytimes.com/2009/09/10/opinion/10pollan.html?mcubz=1.

Chapter 15: One Great Subject

1. J. M. Morgan, "Mālama ʻĀina, Kalo, and Hoʻopili: Growing a Third-Way Environmental Relationship" (PhD diss., University of Hawaiʻi at Manoa, 2016).

2. E. F. Davis, *Scripture, Culture, and Agriculture: An Agrarian Reading of the Bible* (New York: Cambridge University Press, 2009).

3. *The Economist,* "Idea: Triple Bottom Line," *The Economist,* 17 November 2009, www.economist.com/node/14301663.

4. A. C. Newton, D. C. Guy, and K. Preedy, "Wheat Cultivar Yield Response to Some Organic and Conventional Farming Conditions and the Yield Potential of Mixtures," *Journal of Agricultural Science* 155, no. 7 (2017): 1045–60, https://doi.org/10.1017/S002185961700017X.

5. D. Barber, *The Third Plate: Field Notes on the Future of Food* (New York: Penguin Books, 2014).

6. Barber, *Third Plate.*

7. F. Jabr, "Bread Is Broken," *New York Times Magazine,* 29 October 2015, www.nytimes.com/2015/11/01/magazine/bread-is-broken.html?mcubz =1.

8. E. Goldberg, "The Bread Lab Wants to Change the Way We Eat Wheat," *Bon Appétit,* 18 May 2015, www.bonappetit.com/entertaining-style /trends-news/article/bread-lab.

9. A. Eisler, "The Bread Lab: A Growing Partnership," http://thebreadlab .wsu.edu/the-bread-lab-a-growing-partnership/.

10. Jabr, *Bread Is Broken.*

11. Jabr, *Bread Is Broken.*

12. Goldberg, "Bread Lab."

13. Washington State University, College of Agricultural, Human, and Natural Resource Sciences, "About the Bread Lab," http://thebreadlab.wsu .edu/about-the-bread-lab/.

Chapter 16: Rejecting the Status Quo

1. Organic Trade Association, "Organic Purchasing: State-by-State Data Shows Increase in Organic Purchasing throughout U.S.," https://ota.com /resources/organic-purchasing.

2. Organic Trade Association, "Percentage of U.S. Households Purchasing Organic Products," https://ota.com/sites/default/files/indexed_files /HouseholdPenetrationOnly.pdf.

3. Organic Trade Association, "Organic Industry Survey," https://ota.com /resources/organic-industry-survey.

4. US Department of Agriculture, Economic Research Service, "Organic Production: Documentation," 22 September 2016, www.ers.usda.gov /data-products/organic-production/documentation/.

5. M. S. DeLonge, A. Miles, and L. Carlisle, "Investing in the Transition

to Sustainable Agriculture," *Environmental Science & Policy* 55, part 1 (2016): 266–73, https://doi.org/10.1016/j.envsci.2015.09.013.

6. M. Ye et al., "Occupational Pesticide Exposures and Respiratory Health," *International Journal of Environmental Research and Public Health* 10, no. 12 (2013), 6442–71, https://doi.org/10.3390/ijerph10126442; K. Owens, J. Feldman, and J. Kepner, "Wide Range of Diseases Linked to Pesticides," *Pesticides and You* 30, no. 2 (2010): 13–21.

7. E. Simonetti et al., "An Interlaboratory Comparative Study on the Quantitative Determination of Glyphosate at Low Levels in Wheat Flour," *Journal of AOAC International* 98, no. 6 (2015): 1760–68, https://doi.org/10.5740/jaoacint.15-024.

8. Simonetti et al., "Interlaboratory Comparative Study."

9. World Health Organization, International Agency for Research on Cancer, "IARC Monographs Volume 112: Evaluation of Five Organophosphate Insecticides and Herbicides," 20 March 2015, www.iarc.fr/en/media-centre/iarcnews/pdf/MonographVolume112.pdf.

10. US Department of Agriculture, Agricultural Marketing Service, Science and Technology Programs, "Pesticide Data Program: Annual Summary, Calendar Year 2011," app. C, "Distribution of Residues by Pesticide in Soybeans," www.ams.usda.gov/sites/default/files/media/2011%20PDP%20Annual%20Summary.pdf.

11. C. Gillam, "Weedkiller Found in Granola and Crackers, Internal FDA Emails Show," *Guardian* (US edition), 30 April 2018, www.theguardian.com/us-news/2018/apr/30/fda-weedkiller-glyphosate-in-food-internal-emails.

12. A. Leu, *The Myths of Safe Pesticides* (Austin, TX: Acres U.S.A., 2014).

13. A.-M. Klein et al., "Importance of Pollinators in Changing Landscapes for World Crops," *Proceedings of the Royal Society B* 274, no. 1608 (2007): 303–13, https://doi.org/10.1098/rspb.2006.3721.

14. P. Neumann and N. L. Carreck, "Honey Bee Colony Losses," *Journal of Apicultural Research* 49, no. 1 (2010): 1–6, https://doi.org/10.3896/IBRA.1.49.1.01.

15. S. A. Cameron et al., "Patterns of Widespread Decline in North American Bumble Bees," *Proceedings of the National Academy of Sciences of the United States of America* 108, no. 2 (2011): 662–67, https://doi.org/10.1073/pnas.1014743108.

16. R. G. Hatfield et al., *IUCN Assessments for North American Bombus spp.*

for the North American IUCN Bumble Bee Specialist Group (Portland, OR: Xerces Society for Invertebrate Conservation, 2014).

17. S. G. Potts et al., "Global Pollinator Declines: Trends, Impacts, and Drivers," *Trends in Ecology & Evolution* 25, no. 6 (2010): 345–53, https://doi .org/10.1016/j.tree.2010.01.007.

18. D. Goulson, "Review: An Overview of the Environmental Risks Posed by Neonicotinoid Insecticides," *Journal of Applied Ecology* 50, no. 4 (2013): 977–87, https://doi.org/10.1111/1365-2664.12111.

19. I. Heap, "Herbicide Resistant Weeds," in *Integrated Pest Management*, vol. 3, *Pesticide Problems*, ed. D. Pimentel and R. Peshin (Dordrecht: Springer Netherlands, 2014), pp. 281–301.

20. MSU News Service, "MSU Researchers See Troubling Soil Acidity Levels in Montana Agricultural Lands," *Helena (MT) Independent Record*, 6 July 2018, https://helenair.com/news/local/msu-researchers-see-troubling-soil -acidity-levels-in-montana-agricultural/article_e2703c3f-4e3e-5717-8dbb -afa9ee0b244c.html.

21. International Panel of Experts on Sustainable Food Systems (IPES-Food), "From Uniformity to Diversity: A Paradigm Shift from Industrial Agriculture to Diversified Agroecological Systems," June 2016, www.ipes-food .org/images/Reports/UniformityToDiversity_FullReport.pdf.

22. National Oceanic and Atmospheric Administration (NOAA), "Gulf of Mexico 'Dead Zone' Is the Largest Ever Measured," 2 August 2017, www .noaa.gov/media-release/gulf-of-mexico-dead-zone-is-largest-ever-measured.

23. P. K. Thornton, "Recalibrating Food Production in the Developing World: Global Warming Will Change More than Just the Climate," CCAFS Policy Brief No. 6 (Copenhagen: CGIAR Research Program on Climate Change, Agriculture and Food Security, 2012).

24. N. Gilbert, "One-Third of Our Greenhouse Gas Emissions Come from Agriculture," *Nature*, 31 October 2012, https://doi.org/10.1038/nature .2012.11708.

25. E. Aguilera et al., "Managing Soil Carbon for Climate Change Mitigation and Adaptation in Mediterranean Cropping Systems: A Meta-analysis," *Agriculture, Ecosystems & Environment* 168 (2013): 25–36, https://doi.org /10.1016/j.agee.2013.02.003.

26. I. Tomlinson, "Doubling Food Production to Feed the 9 Billion: A Critical Perspective on a Key Discourse of Food Security in the UK," *Journal of Rural Studies* 29 (2013): 81–90, https://doi.org/10.1016/j.jrurstud .2011.09.001; V. Smil, "Improving Efficiency and Reducing Waste in Our

Food System," *Environmental Sciences* 1, no. 1 (2004): 17–26, https://doi.org/10.1076/evms.1.1.17.23766; U. Ramakrishnan, "Prevalence of Micronutrient Malnutrition Worldwide," *Nutrition Reviews* 60, no. S5 (2002): S46–52, https://doi.org/10.1301/00296640260130731.

27. L. C. Smith and L. Haddad, "Reducing Child Undernutrition: Past Drivers and Priorities for the Post-MDG Era," *World Development* 68 (2015): 180–204, https://doi.org/10.1016/j.worlddev.2014.11.014.

28. P. McMichael, "A Food Regime Analysis of the 'World Food Crisis,'" *Agriculture and Human Values* 26 (2009): 281–95, https://doi.org/10.1007/s10460-009-9218-5.

29. K. D. Hall et al., "The Progressive Increase of Food Waste in America and Its Environmental Impact," *PLoS ONE* 4, no. 11 (2009): e7940, https://doi.org/10.1371/journal.pone.0007940; T. Stuart, *Waste: Uncovering the Global Food Scandal* (New York: W. W. Norton, 2009).

30. C. Kremen, "Demand-Side Interventions: A Response to *Breakthrough*'s Essay on Wildlife and Farmland," *Breakthrough*, 28 March 2017, https://thebreakthrough.org/index.php/issues/the-future-of-food/responses-food-production-and-wildlife-on-farmland/demand-side-interventions.

31. Kremen, "Demand-Side Interventions."

32. C. Badgley et al., "Organic Agriculture and the Global Food Supply," *Renewable Agriculture and Food Systems* 22, no. 2 (2007): 86–108, https://doi.org/10.1017/S1742170507001640.

33. L. C. Ponisio et al., "Diversification Practices Reduce Organic to Conventional Yield Gap," *Proceedings of the Royal Society B* 282, no. 1799 (2015), https://doi.org/10.1098/rspb.2014.1396.

34. Kremen, "Demand-Side Interventions."

35. Badgley et al., "Organic Agriculture."

36. V. D. Picasso et al., "Crop Species Diversity Affects Productivity and Weed Suppression in Perennial Polycultures under Two Management Strategies," *Crop Science* 48, no. 1 (2008): 331–42, https://doi.org/10.2135/cropsci2007.04.0225; B. J. Cardinale et al., "Impacts of Plant Diversity on Biomass Production Increase through Time Because of Species Complementarity," *Proceedings of the National Academy of Sciences of the United States of America* 104, no. 46 (2007): 18123–28, https://doi.org/10.1073/pnas.0709069104.

37. J. Pretty, C. Toulmin, and S. Williams, "Sustainable Intensification in African Agriculture," *International Journal of Agricultural Sustainability* 9, no. 1 (2011): 5–24, https://doi.org/10.3763/ijas.2010.0583.

38. F. H. King, *Farmers of Forty Centuries; Or, Permanent Agriculture in China, Korea, and Japan* (London: Butler and Tanner, 1927).

39. D. K. Ray et al., "Recent Patterns of Crop Yield Growth and Stagnation," *Nature Communications* 3 (2012): 1293, https://doi.org/10.1038/ncom ms2296.

40. United Nations Convention to Combat Desertification, "Zero Net Land Degradation—A Sustainable Development Goal for Rio+20: To Secure the Contribution of Our Planet's Land and Soil to Sustainable Development, Including Food Security and Poverty Eradication," UNCCD Secretariat Policy Brief, May 2012, Bonn.

41. D. Butler, "Fungus Threatens Top Banana," *Nature* 504 (12 December 2013): 195–96, https://doi.org/10.1038/504195a; D. Leatherdale, "The Imminent Death of the Cavendish Banana and Why It Affects Us All," *BBC News*, 24 January 2016, www.bbc.com/news/uk-england-35131751.

42. D. W. Lotter, R. Seidel, and W. Lieblardt, "The Performance of Organic and Conventional Cropping Systems in an Extreme Climate Year," *American Journal of Alternative Agriculture* 18, no. 3 (2003): 146–54, https://doi.org/10.1079/AJAA200345; C. Kremen and A. Miles, "Ecosystem Services in Biologically Diversified versus Conventional Farming Systems: Benefits, Externalities, and Trade-Offs," *Ecology and Society* 17, no. 4 (2012): 40, http://dx.doi.org/10.5751/ES-05035-170440.

43. A. D. Jones, A. Shrinivas, and R. Bezner-Kerr, "Farm Production Diversity Is Associated with Greater Household Dietary Diversity in Malawi: Findings from Nationally Representative Data," *Food Policy* 46 (2014) 1–12, https://doi.org/10.1016/j.foodpol.2014.02.001.

44. G. Carletto et al., "Farm-Level Pathways to Improved Nutritional Status: Introduction to the Special Issue," *Journal of Development Studies* 51, no. 8 (2015): 945–57, https://doi.org/10.1080/00220388.2015.1018908.

45. M. Barański et al., "Higher Antioxidant and Lower Cadmium Concentrations and Lower Incidence of Pesticide Residues in Organically Grown Crops: A Systematic Literature Review and Meta-analyses," *British Journal of Nutrition* 112, no. 5 (2014): 794–811, https://doi.org/10.1017/S000 7114514001366.

46. G. Schütte et al., "Herbicide Resistance and Biodiversity: Agronomic and Environmental Aspects of Genetically Modified Herbicide-Resistant Plants," *Environmental Sciences Europe* 29, no. 1 (2017): 5, http://doi.org/10.1186/s12302-016-0100-y.

47. B. Hoffman, "GMO Crops Mean More Herbicide, Not Less," *Forbes*, 2

July 2013, www.forbes.com/sites/bethhoffman/2013/07/02/gmo-crops
-mean-more-herbicide-not-less/#2b6a35f93cd5.

48. D. Hakim, "Doubts about the Promised Bounty of Genetically Modified Crops," *New York Times*, 29 October 2016, www.nytimes.com/2016/10 /30/business/gmo-promise-falls-short.html.

49. US Department of Agriculture, National Agricultural Statistics Service, "Agricultural Chemical Use Program," 2010, www.nass.usda.gov/Surveys /Guide_to_NASS_Surveys/Chemical_Use/.

Chapter 17: Conclusion: A New Generation of Growers and Eaters

1. M. B. Marcus, "The Top 10 Leading Causes of Death in the U.S.," *CBS News*, 30 June 2016, www.cbsnews.com/news/the-leading-causes-of -death-in-the-us/; W. C. Willett, "Balancing Life-Style and Genomics Research for Disease Prevention," *Science* 296, no. 5568 (26 April 2002): 695–98, http://doi.org/10.1126/science.1071055; M. Pollan, *In Defense of Food: An Eater's Manifesto* (New York: Penguin Books, 2008), p. 136.

2. S. Jayaraman, "To Fight Harassment in Restaurants, We Must Start with Wages," *Food & Wine*, 20 November 2017, www.foodandwine.com/news /sexual-harassment-restaurant-industry-wage-system.

3. Associated Press, "Farm Population Lowest since 1850's," *New York Times*, 20 July 1988, www.nytimes.com/1988/07/20/us/farm-population-lowest -since-1850-s.html.

4. R. Hayden-Smith, *Sowing the Seeds of Victory: American Gardening Programs of World War I* (Jefferson, NC: McFarland & Company, 2014), http://rosehayden-smith.com/fruits-victory-stats/.

5. R. B. Reich, *Aftershock: The Next Economy and America's Future* (New York: Knopf, 2010).

6. W. Hauter, *Foodopoly: The Battle over the Future of Food and Farming in America* (New York: New Press, 2012), p. 22.

7. E. Schlosser, *Fast Food Nation: The Dark Side of the All-American Meal* (New York: Penguin Books, 2002).

8. E. Barclay, "Your Grandparents Spent More of Their Money on Food than You Do," *The Salt*, National Public Radio, 2 March 2015, www.npr .org/sections/thesalt/2015/03/02/389578089/your-grandparents-spent -more-of-their-money-on-food-than-you-do.

9. T. McMillan, "Food Workers Scramble to Put Food on Their Tables," *The Plate* (blog), *National Geographic*, 14 November 2016, https://www .nationalgeographic.com/people-and-culture/food/the-plate/2016/11 /food-workers-find-it-hard-to-put-food-on-their-tables/.

10. S. Jayaraman, "It's Been Twenty-Five Years since Restaurant Workers Got a Raise," *Talk Poverty*, 1 April 2016, https://talkpoverty.org/2016/04/01/25-years-since-restauraunt-workers-got-a-raise/.

11. D. Pimentel et al., "Environmental, Energetic, and Economic Comparisons of Organic and Conventional Farming Systems," *BioScience* 55, no. 7 (2005): 573–82, https://doi.org/10.1641/0006-3568(2005)055[0573:EEAECO]2.0.CO;2.

12. D. Eller, "With Water Works' Lawsuit Dismissed, Water Quality Is the Legislature's Problem," *Des Moines Register*, 17 March 2017, www.desmoinesregister.com/story/money/agriculture/2017/03/17/judge-dismisses-water-works-nitrates-lawsuit/99327928/.

13. "The Healthcare Costs of Obesity," *State of Obesity*, https://stateofobesity.org/healthcare-costs-obesity/.

14. Pollan, *In Defense of Food*, pp. 187–88.

15. O. Khazan, "Why Are So Many Americans Dying Young?," *The Atlantic*, 13 December 2016, www.theatlantic.com/health/archive/2016/12/why-are-so-many-americans-dying-young/510455/; D. Ludwig, "Declining Life Expectancy According to New CDC Data," *Medium*, 4 April 2016, https://medium.com/@davidludwigmd/declining-life-expectancy-according-to-new-cdc-data-d137ae07d1bb.

16. J. Kell, "Soda Consumption Falls to 30-Year Low in the U.S.," *Fortune*, 29 March 2016, http://fortune.com/2016/03/29/soda-sales-drop-11th-year/.

17. Centers for Disease Control and Prevention, "Current Cigarette Smoking among Adults in the United States," 2018, www.cdc.gov/tobacco/data_statistics/fact_sheets/adult_data/cig_smoking/index.htm; L. Saad, "U.S. Smoking Rate Still Coming Down," *Gallup News*, 24 July 2008, https://news.gallup.com/poll/109048/us-smoking-rate-still-coming-down.aspx.

18. N. Bakalar, "Americans Are Putting Down the Soda Pop," *New York Times*, 14 November 2017, www.nytimes.com/2017/11/14/health/soda-pop-sugary-drinks.html.

19. L. Nargi, "Is a Federal Junk Food Tax in Our Future?," *Civil Eats*, 11 January 2018, https://civileats.com/2018/01/11/is-a-federal-junk-food-tax-in-our-future/.

20. M. Pollan, "How Change Is Going to Come in the Food System," *The Nation*, 14 September 2011, www.thenation.com/article/how-change-going-come-food-system/.

21. K. Klein, "Values-Based Food Procurement in Hospitals: The Role of

Health Care Group Purchasing Organizations," *Agriculture and Human Values* 32, no. 4 (2015): 635–48, https://doi.org/10.1007/s10460-015 -9586-y.

22. D. Miller, "A Doctor Takes a Closer Look at How Nutrition Might Help Her Patients," *Washington Post*, 26 May 2009, www.washingtonpost.com /wp-dyn/content/article/2009/05/22/AR2009052202280.html.

23. Klein, "Values-Based Food Procurement."

24. The Nielsen Company, "Green Generation: Millennials Say Sustainability Is a Shopping Priority," 5 November 2015, www.nielsen.com/us/en /insights/news/2015/green-generation-millennials-say-sustainability-is -a-shopping-priority.html.

25. P. Cantrell, "Sysco's Journey from Supply Chain to Value Chain," August 2009, www.ngfn.org/resources/research-1/innovative-models/NGFN%20 Case%20Study_Syscos%20Journey%20From%20Supply%20Chain%20 to%20Value%20Chain.pdf.

26. C. Dewey, "A Growing Number of Young Americans Are Leaving Desk Jobs to Farm," *Washington Post*, 23 November 2017, www.washington post.com/business/economy/a-growing-number-of-young-americans-are -leaving-desk-jobs-to-farm/2017/11/23/e3c018ae-c64e-11e7-afe9-4f60b 5a6c4a0_story.html?utm_term=.b6903b6b4fe2.

27. J. E. Warnert, "Local Food Movement Drives Interest in Home Food Preservation," *ANR News Blog* (Agriculture and Natural Resources, University of California), 3 February 2016, http://ucanr.edu/blogs/blogcore /postdetail.cfm?postnum=20120; D. L. Spurrier, "Cultivating Interest in the Art of Canning," 4 August 2015, University of Maryland, College of Agriculture & Natural Resources, https://agnr.umd.edu/news/cultivating -interest-art-canning.

Index

cover crops, 57, 62–65, 203
Cowgill, Jacob, 203
cytokines, 184–85, 187, 192

Dave's Killer Bread, 117
Davis, Don, 130
Davis, William, 179–80, 191
DDT, 32
debt, 41
Des Moines Water Works, 223
diabetes, 3, 173, 189–90, 194
Diamond v. Chakrabarty, 85
dicamba, 30–31, 212, 218
diesel fuel, 144–45
dilution effect, 130–31, 136
Dilworth, Thomas, 165–66
disease. *See* health and disease, human
Dow, 116
doxorubicin ("dox"), 177–78
drought
    chemical inputs and, 53, 55
    corn yields during, 217
    cover crops and, 64
    grasshoppers and, 60
    organic experiment and, 59
drought tolerance, 90–91
dryland vegetable farming, 125–31
DuPont, 116

Earthbound Farms, 111
eaters, power of, 229–30
Egypt, 102–3, 106
An Egyptian Hieroglyphic Dictionary
    (Budge), 83–84
einkorn, 106
Elkington, John, 198
endosperm, 49
energy and fuels
    camelina oil, 145–47
    canola oil, 145
    conversion of oil to biodiesel, 146

diesel, 144–45
fossil fuel consumption, 143–45
fuel production vs. food production and,
    152
high-oleic safflower oil, 149–54
wind farms, 154–60
enrichment of white bread, 50–51
environmental impact and carbon
    footprint, 104, 144
epidemiological studies, 173
epigenetics, 190–91
European markets for Kamut wheat,
    95–97, 99–101, 109

family farms, loss of, 39–40
Farm Bureau, 20–21, 22–23, 53, 69
farm crisis, period of, 53
Farmers Union, 20–21, 27
farming. *See specific topics, such as* organic
    farming
Farm Journal, 26
fatty liver disease, nonalcoholic, 190
fertilizer, synthetic
    in Big Sandy, MT, 23
    carbon footprint of, 104, 144
    consequences of, 54–55
    in Egypt, 102–3
    excess, 6
    Haber-Bosch process, 54
    natural vs., 53
    nutrient dilution from, 131
    runoff and pollution from, 9, 212
    soil acidification from, 212
fiber, 173
Finch, Ian, 149–52
flour
    bleaching and enrichment of, 49–51
    stone-ground, 74–75, 173
Flowers Foods, 117
food insecurity, 124, 213–14
food miles, 104